## ALSO BY JJ VIRGIN

*Six Weeks to Sleeveless and Sexy*

*The Virgin Diet Cookbook*

*JJ Virgin's Sugar Impact Diet*

*JJ Virgin's Sugar Impact Diet Cookbook*

# THE VIRGIN DIET

**DROP 7 FOODS, LOSE 7 POUNDS, JUST 7 DAYS**

## JJ VIRGIN, CNS, CHFS

WILLIAM MORROW

*An Imprint of* HarperCollins*Publishers*

The health advice presented in this book is intended only as an informative resource guide to help you make informed decisions; it is not meant to replace the advice of a physician or to serve as a guide to self-treatment. Always seek competent medical help for any health condition or if there is any question about the appropriateness of a procedure or health recommendation.

HarperCollins books may be purchased for educational, business, or sales promotional use. For information please e-mail the Special Markets Department at SPsales@harpercollins.com.

A hardcover edition of this book was published in 2012 by Harlequin Enterprises, Ltd.

FIRST WILLIAM MORROW PAPERBACK EDITION PUBLISHED 2015.

Library of Congress Cataloging-in-Publication Data has been applied for.

ISBN 978-0-06-240679-8

23 24 25 26 27  LBC  12 11 10 9 8

This book is dedicated to frustrated dieters everywhere who have been diligently eating those "healthy foods" and figuring that they were just doomed to be overweight. May this book set you free.

# CONTENTS

# CONTENTS

# ACKNOWLEDGMENTS

So much synchronicity went into the development of this book!

First, I want to thank the amazing science team at Metametrix Clinical Laboratory who helped me realize the impact of low-grade food reactions. I was so fortunate to be able to educate doctors throughout the country on how food sensitivities could be causing a myriad of health issues and then see the side effect that pulling these foods out had on their patients' health: rapid weight loss! I kept seeing the same food reactions coming up over and over again, along with the same benefits, which helped me realize that this was a powerful weight-loss tool!

I want to shout out to Chef Leanne Ely, who tracked me down on Twitter. When I told her about how I pulled people off these foods but couldn't find good recipes for them, she jumped right in and developed them, proving deliciously that cooking and eating this way could be done!

To my pals at Discovery, TLC and Shed Media, it was a blast working with you on *Freaky Eaters*, and I am thrilled to be a part of *Transformation Diaries*. Dr. Mike Dow, I hope we get to be the dream team again sometime soon, and thanks for the amazing hookup to Celeste Fine! Andrew Strauser, you are my casting angel—I so appreciate your continuing to find these amazing opportunities for me. And to my manager, Greg Horangic, thank you for making the deals happen!

To my brilliant literary agent, Celeste Fine, you convinced me that this was the book and made it all happen, from hooking me up with my incredible writing partner, Rachel Kranz, to bringing me to the team at Harlequin, who I fell in love with from the moment I walked in the door. I felt like I had come home! I feel so fortunate to be working with my amazing editor, Sarah Pelz, and the whole team at Harlequin has been incredible. I am so honored that you chose me.

Big kudos to my publicist extraordinaire, Barbara Teszler, for helping me get the message out to millions. You are the pitch genius. Mike Danielson at Media Relations, you are brilliant with your connections and ideas. And Jason Boehm, thanks for stalking me—what did I do before you? You are not only my social media genius but also my second set of eyes into all that is going on in our world. To my attorney, Darryl Sheetz, thanks for always having my back and keeping me safe out there in the business world!

I am supported everyday by an incredible team at www.jjvirgin.com. Susan Tafralis, you are my rock and my number-one support system; I couldn't do it without you. Thanks to Mary Ann Guillory, who keeps me in line with my shoe habit and makes sure the money is flowing in the right direction; to Traci Knoppe, who handles all things technical; Patsy Wallace and Jason Boehm, my rock star health coaches; and Julia Zaslow, who is an absolute genius in marketing and strategy.

Another big shout-out to all of those who help me continue to nurture my business, including my current business coach, the amazing Brendon Burchard. I feel so blessed to be working with you. Dr. Daniel Amen, you are my role model and so genuine and generous—I adore you. And thanks to Ali Brown for opening my eyes to the power of the online world as my first real business coach and one of my dearest friends. Thanks also to Lisa Sasevich for teaching me how to package and position my work so people will take action. To my sweet friend Marcelle Pick of Women to Women, your work on stress and food sensitivities was so helpful in putting this book together. Kaayla Daniel, thanks for jumping in at the 11th hour with brilliant information. A huge thank-you to Hooman "the great" Fakki of H2 Wellness. Suzanne Somers, of course I have to include you here, as your courageous work continues to pave the way for all of us. To all of my amazing and courageous pals in the integrative health field who are getting the word out there and taking the bullets for "going against the grain," you are all such inspiration and support for me.

And finally to my sons, Grant and Bryce: Thank you for your patience, support and love. You are ultimately why I am doing all of this. You are my "inspired why." I feel so blessed to be your mom. John Virgin, thanks for being there to let me do what I needed to do to make it all happen. I so appreciate you. And to my mommy, I know you still aren't totally sure about what I do (besides travel *a lot*), but don't worry, I have a great boss who won't be firing me anytime soon! Thanks for setting me up to be the strong, confident woman I am.

## How the Virgin Diet Can Change Your Life

Melanie was a 40-year-old brand manager who had been struggling with her weight for the past 15 years. She was the classic yo-yo dieter, always losing the same 10 pounds and then always gaining it back. Lately, though, she had started gaining back more than she lost, first an extra 15 pounds, then an extra 20. When she came to me, she was beyond frustrated—and not at all sure that I could help her.

"Look," she told me during our first consultation, "I know what you're going to say, but please don't say it. I don't binge. I do watch what I eat. I count every calorie I put into my mouth. Yes, I eat in restaurants occasionally, but I always have just a salad or maybe some broiled fish. I live on low-fat, low-carb foods, I never let myself have dessert, I exercise five times a week and I don't even drink! But here I am, 20 pounds overweight, bursting out of my clothes and my skin is breaking out. I'm just a mess."

"Okay," I said, thinking that Melanie was just the kind of client I love to work with. Like me, she was a no-nonsense gal who didn't waste time, and I knew she would respond well to my particular brand of "tough love—with love."

"Just answer three questions," I said. "First, do you drink milk or eat yogurt?"

"Every day," she said proudly. "Nonfat only, of course."

"What about eggs, including egg whites? Ever have those in your diet?"

"Every day," she repeated.

"And soy—tofu, soy sauce, edamame—is that something you eat as well?"

"Every day," she said a third time, awaiting her gold star.

"Okay, so here's the problem, Melanie. A lot of these so-called healthy foods are actually not good for you. And believe it or not, they can cause you to gain weight."

We were having a phone consultation, so I couldn't see Melanie's face, but I could imagine her surprise because I've seen it on the faces of thousands of people I've worked with—the weight-loss clients I advise, the health care professionals I speak to, the physicians I help to educate about diet and nutrition. Sometimes I think it's America's best kept secret: *Supposedly healthy foods can actually cause you to gain weight.*

"The problem," I explained to Melanie, "is a condition known as food intolerance."

"Wait a minute," Melanie said, interrupting me. "Are you telling me I'm allergic to food?"

Even though Melanie couldn't see me, I shook my head. "Food allergies are a very specific condition. They're one type of immune system response—usually very fast and very intense. Food intolerance is usually slower and more subtle. It's an umbrella term that covers a lot of different ways that your body might have trouble digesting food."

I explained to Melanie that sometimes *food intolerance* (FI) is a preexisting condition. You might have been born intolerant to certain foods, such as dairy products or gluten—a protein found in many grains, breads, pastas and baked goods, as well as in many processed and prepared foods. Or you might have developed food intolerance later in your life. Sometimes it's set off by stress, which disrupts your body's functioning in several different ways. You might have developed food intolerance from eating too much of the same food every day. If this is a food that your body is reacting to, it can lead to a buildup of immune complexes that set off a myriad of symptoms. Food intolerance might result from many other causes, including a condition known as leaky gut, which itself can be set off by infection, antibiotics, radiation, heavy metals and a host of other causes, including, again, stress. (We'll look more at the causes of food intolerance in Chapter 1.)

In some cases, food intolerance is permanent. There may just be some foods that will present you with lifelong problems. Fortunately, in many cases, food intolerance can be overcome. If you stay away from a food long enough and repair your system with healing foods and supplements, you might be able to tolerate the problematic food later on.

"So," I told Melanie, "if food intolerance is *your* problem—and it certainly sounds as though it might be—there is a quick, simple solution. All you have to do is drop the top 7 *high-FI foods*—the 7 foods most likely to cause food intolerance. In 7 days, you can lose up to 7 pounds and look years younger. What do you say?"

Melanie might have been surprised, but she didn't let it slow her down. "Absolutely," she said, as quickly as I'd thought she might. "Let's get started."

## FOOD INTOLERANCE: THE HIDDEN CAUSE OF WEIGHT GAIN

If you wanted to be your skinniest self and follow the healthiest diet in the world, what would you eat? Egg-white veggie omelets? Greek-style nonfat yogurt? Low-calorie whey protein shakes? A soy-based veggie burger on a whole-grain bun?

That sounds like the regimen that famous trainers and A-list stars follow, doesn't it? But what if I told you that I've been a sought-after fitness and nutrition expert for over 2 decades and worked with thousands of clients, including some of Hollywood's hottest bodies? And what if I told you what I told them, which is that many of these supposedly healthy foods could actually be making you fat?

Well, that's exactly what I am going to tell you. So listen up, because I'm about to share with you the secret to weight loss.

It isn't calories.

It isn't fat.

It isn't protein.

It isn't even carbs.

Sure, those things can be important. But you can count them, cut them, skinny them and swap them all you want, and you won't lose weight if you're eating foods that your body can't handle.

> **You won't lose weight if you're eating foods that your body can't handle.**

*The key to weight loss is avoiding and overcoming food intolerance.*

Food intolerance is a series of physiological responses that your body has to certain types of food. They aren't the same as allergies. Most people test negative for food allergies, but most people have at least one type of food intolerance, and many have several.

Food-intolerance symptoms vary from person to person, but the most common include bloating, gas, indigestion, fatigue, mental fog, irritability, moodiness—and weight gain. If you're eating foods that your body can't tolerate, you're likely to gain weight, feel crummy and look years older than your actual age.

Most people ignore their bodies' responses to the foods they eat, or maybe they search for ways to mask the symptoms. But weight gain, bloating and fatigue are not just annoying facts of life. They are your body's way of telling you that you're eating foods that aren't working for you. Until you get rid of the foods that your body can't handle, load up on healing foods and supplements and give your body a chance to recover from what you've unknowingly put it through, you are likely to gain weight, retain weight and suffer from premature aging. Not a pretty picture.

Maybe your body is stressed because of your daily diet's high content of sugar, artificial sweeteners and processed foods, which tend to contain lots of high-FI soy, corn and gluten. Or perhaps you've maintained a seemingly healthy natural, low-fat and low-carb regime but have never realized that all of your healthy efforts are being sabotaged by high-FI yogurt (even nonfat), eggs (even omega-3–rich) and grains (even whole). Either way, if you weigh more than you'd like and look older than you'd prefer, you are most likely struggling with food intolerances.

How can you tell? Let me ask you what I ask my clients:

- Have you tried unsuccessfully to lose weight?
- Is what you used to do to lose weight no longer working?
- Are you a yo-yo dieter?
- Do you frequently experience discomfort after eating, such as bloating, gas or indigestion?
- Can you only lose weight by starving yourself or exercising like a maniac—or possibly not even then?
- Are you feeling and looking older than you should?

If the answer to even one of these questions is yes, you've likely been eating too many *high-FI foods:* problem foods that are likely to trigger food intolerance. What's the solution? Stop eating high-FI foods and replace them with *low-FI foods:* foods that are unlikely to trigger food intolerance. If you can cut out the top 7 high-FI foods for just 3 weeks, you'll see weight loss and beauty results that will have you looking and feeling terrific.

Hey, if those old low-fat, low-carb or high-protein diets had worked for you in the past, you'd already be at your ideal weight and peak vitality, right? There's a reason that approach to food doesn't work—and there's a reason that the Virgin Diet does.

## YOUR FAT IS NOT YOUR FAULT

I often joke that most of my clients are allergic to diets. And in a way, they are, because most of the foods that people eat when they diet—egg whites, nonfat yogurt, tofu—can set off food intolerance that keeps the weight on, even when you cut the calories.

The "allergic" part is my joke, because food intolerance and food allergies are not actually the same thing. However, they are very closely related. They're both responses to an apparently harmless or maybe even a healthy food that can involve one or more of your body's systems, including your digestive system and your immune system. High-FI foods not only make you feel tired, unfocused and moody, but they're also the hidden cause of weight gain, weight-loss resistance and premature aging.

The good news here is that your fat is not your fault. It's your body's way of responding to the foods it can't handle—foods you may have been eating precisely because you thought they were good for you!

Luckily, there is a solution: the three-week Virgin Diet solution. For just 21 days:

- Stop eating the 7 major high-FI foods.
- Focus on low-FI foods that will give your digestive system a break.

- Load up with healing foods and healing supplements to repair the damage.

Right away, you'll lose the bloat, finally start losing weight and look years younger. You'll look and feel so terrific that you might even make some lifelong changes in your diet.

## THE TOP 7 HIGH-FI FOODS

| | | |
|---|---|---|
| Gluten | Eggs | Sugar and Artificial Sweeteners |
| Soy | Corn | |
| Dairy | Peanuts | |

## HOW ELIMINATING HIGH-FI FOODS FIGHTS THE POUNDS—AND THE YEARS

Food intolerance isn't a fixed condition; it's more like a dynamic response. Foods that you were able to tolerate a few years ago might be problematic for you now. If you clean high-FI foods out of your system and take some other healing steps—all of which I'll walk you through—then you may eventually be able to eat foods that are causing problems for you now.

The first step, though, is to get those high-FI foods out of your system and give your body a chance to chill out. After a 21-day break, I'll have you add some of the healthier high-FI foods back into your diet, and we'll find out if you can tolerate them. If you can't handle them right away, you may be able to in 3 months, or 6 months or perhaps a year. But before we can add them back in, we have to take them out.

A lot of my clients are skeptical about this elimination process, at least at first. They just can't believe that such apparently healthy foods as yogurt, whole grains and edamame are causing such severe problems, especially when they don't cause any noticeable ill effects after eating them. That's because food intolerance is such a subtle reaction. Allergies are swifter and more dramatic. A peanut allergy can strike after one tiny bite of peanut. Your throat closes up, you can hardly breathe and the conclusion is pretty clear: stay away from peanuts.

Food intolerance is sneakier. If you enjoy a delicious bowl of non-fat yogurt and berries today and break out in acne 2 days later, you're unlikely to make the connection—but I'm betting that it's there. (See Chapter 5 for more information on the strong link between dairy and acne.) Likewise, if you have some whole-grain cereal this morning, you might not even realize that it's the cause of your fitful sleep tonight. You probably *won't* realize it until you eliminate gluten for a few weeks and start sleeping like a baby.

Like I said, high-FI foods are sneaky. They work slowly, subtly and after long delays. The only way to find out how they're affecting you is to cut them out for at least 21 days. If your skin clears up, your hair perks up and your energy levels rise, maybe we're onto something here. And if you drop up to 7 pounds in 7 days, I think you might say that we've figured out your problem.

Allergy specialists are quite familiar with elimination diets: food regimens in which a possibly offending food is removed from your diet and then gradually reintroduced a few weeks later. If you can introduce the problem food easily, then you either weren't allergic to it or you've gotten past the allergy. If reintroduction causes symptoms to flare up, then you've found a food that your body can't handle, at least not right now.

The Virgin Diet works the same way. We take out the foods that might be causing you problems. We will then reintroduce some high-FI foods—eggs, dairy, soy and gluten—back into your diet. If you tolerate them well, terrific! If you show symptoms, out they go. You can give them another try in 3, 6 or 12 months when your system has had more time to heal and recover. I am going to encourage you to keep the sugar, artificial sweeteners, corn and peanuts out of your diet for the long haul (or at least 95 percent

> You can do just about anything for 21 days.

of the time), but let's deal with that once you recognize how amazing you feel without them! Right now, just focus on the fact that this is only for 21 days. And you can do just about anything for 21 days.

For our first step, the key is to avoid moderation. We need literally zero quantities of gluten, soy, dairy, eggs, corn, peanuts, sugar and artificial sweeteners. That's the only way to stop stressing your system.

What are the benefits of temporarily eliminating high-FI foods?

1. **Relief of symptoms.** Many of my clients never even realized they had symptoms until they cut out the high-FI foods. Perhaps your "normal" is to feel exhausted, stressed out, cranky and hungry, and you think it's because you're scrambling to meet deadlines, stressing over your parents and fighting with your boyfriend. Maybe . . . or maybe your life feels so out of control because high-FI foods are undermining your ability to sleep deeply, concentrate well and handle difficulties with good, calm energy. I'm betting that cutting out the high-FI foods will bring you to a whole new normal: energized, cheerful, calm and satisfied. If dropping high-FI foods made you feel that good,

would you do it? What if you could finally lose that extra weight and look 10 years younger as well?

2. **Rapid weight loss and antiaging benefits.** Even if you're not experiencing symptoms, high-FI foods are almost certainly behind your struggles with weight loss. And if you feel that you're looking older and more tired than you'd like, there's a strong possibility that high-FI foods are the culprit. Drop the high-FI foods, drop up to 7 pounds in 7 days and look years younger. That's my promise, and I can't wait for you to take me up on it.

If you eliminate a high-FI food and then reintroduce it, you'll know instantly if it's been causing you trouble because any symptoms you have will be through the roof. I had a client who had never realized that she'd been struggling with egg intolerance. When she cut out eggs, she lost 10 pounds in 3 weeks without even trying. Then, when she ate an experimental plate of scrambled eggs, she got so sleepy that she almost passed out. Eggs had been making her tired, fat and old before her time. It was only when she gave them up that she figured it out.

Have you ever heard the story of the lobster who didn't realize it was being cooked because the water just kept on getting warmer and warmer? That's how a lot of my clients are about eating high-FI foods. That's how I was, too. One day I woke up and realized that I had gained 10 pounds, had developed a bloated waistline and was struggling with mental fog and fatigue almost all the time. I hate to admit it, but I also looked 10 years older. How had this happened? My symptoms had developed gradually, and I had simply learned to live with them.

When I cut out high-FI foods, my new normal was terrific. I lost all the weight I had gained, and I looked young and glowing again. Problem solved, right? Then I took one tiny bite of egg—by accident, it was lurking in a sauce—and I almost doubled over with cramps and bloating. Suddenly it looked like an alien was growing in my stomach.

The Virgin Diet is the key to losing those stubborn pounds—and all those extra years. If I want to keep feeling good, looking young and staying slim, I stick to the Virgin Diet. Now you can follow the Virgin Diet and get the same great results.

# YOUR FAT IS NOT YOUR FATE

Like most people, you've probably longed for your old figure and your younger metabolism. You've chalked up your leaner friends' skinny jeans to luck and genetics. You've tried every fad diet and superfood, hoping to resemble the Hollywood stars who look better at 40 than they did at 20, seemingly by magic. And you are reluctantly accepting a fate of an ever-expanding waistline as part of aging.

Well, what if I told you that fat is not your fate? I'm almost 50 years old, and I put most younger women's bodies to shame. Better yet, so do my clients. You can stop gaining weight and lose the pounds you've packed on over the last decade simply by eliminating the bad foods. Time makes you wiser not wider, and you have probably spent a lifetime of moderately consuming the wrong foods and gradually undermining your body's ability to maintain or lose weight. The fewer wrong foods you eat, the leaner you will be. By eliminating all the wrong foods for 3 weeks, you can drop up to 7 pounds and look years younger by next week.

> You can stop gaining weight and lose the pounds simply by eliminating the bad foods.

Let's get one thing straight: even if you've been on a dozen diets and struggled unsuccessfully to lose weight, the Virgin Diet can work for you. In fact, the more trouble you've had with losing weight and keeping it off, the more likely it is that food intolerance is at the root of your problem. Ironically, trouble with previous diets probably makes you a better candidate for success with the Virgin Diet. If they didn't work, food intolerance was very likely a big part of the reason. Heal that problem, and off come the pounds.

> The more trouble you've had losing weight, the more likely it is that food intolerance is your problem.

Does pulling high-FI foods from your diet sound like an impossible task? Believe me, I get it. I hated the thought of giving up my favorite high-FI foods. I wondered how I'd live without my occasional slice of sourdough bread and my beloved breakfast omelets. I couldn't believe I'd ever be happy without that inch of foamy milk on my cafè Americano. The irony is that you usually crave the very foods that are hurting you, and eat them every day.

But you know what? Now that I live on a low-FI diet, I feel happier, healthier and more energetic than I ever have. My mind is clear and focused, and I love the way I look. My life has been much easier to navigate without high-FI foods, and I promise, yours will be, too. In just 3 weeks, you'll reverse your weight gain. You'll look and feel at least 10 years younger. And you'll be able to safely reintroduce the foods that your body likes.

The Virgin Diet can work anywhere with anybody, no matter where you live, how often you eat in restaurants or how frequently you travel. I travel a lot of the time and rarely have time to cook, but when I'm home, I like to make dinner for my kids. I'm not the Queen of Cooking, but I am the Queen of Meal Assembly. I've stuck to the Virgin Diet everywhere in the United States, including some tiny towns too small to even have a full-sized grocery store.

In Part III of this book, I'll show you how to create delicious low-FI meals (including plenty of easy, crowd-pleasing recipes) and how to maintain the diet when you travel, eat in restaurants or cook for your family—even for picky eaters! You can prepare low-FI foods for your family, and you can prepare them on a budget. You don't need access to special health-food stores and you don't need to eat weird or unusual foods. All you have to do is cut the wrong foods out of your diet and replace them with the foods your body likes.

So don't worry about sticking to this program. Whatever your situation, I know you can make it work. Just give me 21 days, and you are going to be blown away by how great you feel.

## THE VIRGIN DIET: YOUR KEY TO WEIGHT LOSS SUCCESS

I've been working with weight loss and food intolerance for more than 20 years. I've helped hundreds of physicians expand their knowledge of nutrition and weight loss, and I've helped thousands of men and women lose weight. Some of my greatest success stories can be found throughout this book. Clients who have struggled with their weight for years suddenly begin losing weight almost without effort—as long as they leave high-FI foods out of their diets. People who have suffered from acne, arthritis, joint pain, mental fog, fatigue and a dozen other complaints suddenly lose their symptoms. Their skin clears up, their hair looks shiny and full of life and they appear 10 years younger. That is their success story—and it can be yours.

It was certainly Melanie's. After 21 days on the Virgin Diet, she lost 10 of her target 20 pounds without any reduction in calories or change to her exercise routine. A few weeks later, she lost the other 10 pounds and was feeling stronger and more energized than she had in years. She no longer had to stress over calorie-counting or obsess over the scale. She just had to leave out of her diet the foods that her body couldn't tolerate.

"You know, it's funny, JJ," she said the last time we talked, "now my friends all want to know what I'm eating to look so terrific."

"That's great," I answered. "What do you tell them?"

Melanie laughed. "I tell them it's what I'm *not* eating that's made all the difference!"

# HOW THE VIRGIN DIET WORKED FOR ME

My problems with weight go back to when I was about 6 or 7 years old, thinking I was fat. I started dieting when I was about 13 years old. My mom took me to the doctor for diet pills when I was 16 years old.

Over the years, I've tried just about every diet known to man, but the weight kept creeping on. Every time, it was the same: I would lose a few pounds and gain it all back plus some. At 40, I weighed more than 315 pounds. I knew I had to change my life, but I wasn't happy, and I found comfort in food. And I had a lot of medical problems. First, I suffered from a pinched ulnar nerve. Then at age 42, I was diagnosed with attention

Kathy Miller
Age 56

Lakewood,
Colorado

**Height:**
5'8"

**Starting Weight:**
298 pounds

**Waist:** 49.5"
**Hips:** 59"

**Current Weight:**
273.2 pounds

**Waist:** 41"
**Hips:** 55"

**Lost:** 24.8 pounds

deficit disorder, or ADD. A couple years later, I was diagnosed with asthma. After years of being hospitalized for asthma attacks and gaining 80 pounds, thanks to medication and depression, I was told by my pulmonary doctor that I had gastroesophageal reflux disease, or GERD, which was exacerbating my asthma. This was the first time I realized that the foods that were causing me to be fat might also be the foods causing these other serious illnesses and disorders.

By this time I was back up to 298 pounds and housebound. I was so fat! I was embarrassed to be seen. I felt like a complete failure. I was on three daily medicines for asthma, a nightly antacid, an ointment for eczema and bottles of ibuprofen for joint pains. I had to wrap an elastic bandage around my knee every day to manage the pain.

When I tried to diet, the results were frustrating until I read about JJ's Virgin Diet. Her explanation of food intolerances described everything I was feeling. I took the symptoms test and marked almost everything with the highest score. Right then, I committed to the plan. After just 3 weeks, I lost 11 pounds, including a couple inches off my waist and hips. I cleaned up my shopping, my kitchen and my health. As it turns out, I am gluten- and dairy-intolerant. And much of the food I thought was healthy really wasn't.

I learned how much I have poisoned my body over the years. Now I don't have cravings for sweets; fast foods; or fatty, starchy, high-carb foods. I am satisfied with whole, clean, natural foods. My asthma symptoms are so much less than before that I almost don't need the medicine at all. My eczema spots are all but gone now. I can take walks without pain. I don't have headaches. I have not had any indigestion since my second day on the plan. My ADD seems to be nonexistent. No more brain fog. No depression. I have energy that I haven't had in years. Most of all, I have *hope*.

I have learned for the first time what to eat, why to eat and when to eat. I feel so much better! This program saved my life!

# HOW "DIET" FOODS ARE MAKING YOU FAT

# FOOD INTOLERANCE

## The Hidden Cause of Weight Gain

Leslie was at the end of her rope. She'd been to every doctor in the Los Angeles area, and nobody could help her. As it happens, her stepmother is Suzanne Somers, an expert in health, beauty and fitness. Suzanne knows all the gurus, besides being one herself. But none of them could fix Leslie's problem. Leslie was 40 pounds overweight. It didn't seem to matter whether she ate or not. She had this chronic bloating thing going on—in fact, she got more and more bloated as the day continued, no matter how little she ate.

I loved Leslie on the spot. She's adorable. And I was struck by how much she was already doing the right things—and how little any of them were helping her.

"What's going on, JJ?" Leslie asked me. At this point, she was beyond frustrated. "You've got to help me out, because nobody else has ever been able to."

I felt a lot of sympathy for Leslie, who was working so hard to lose weight—and with so little result. She exercised and was very careful about counting calories and controlling portions. But as I tell all of my clients, your body isn't a savings bank or a calorimeter. It's a chemistry lab. Counting calories and measuring portions just isn't enough. You have to know how your body is responding to the foods you eat. And Leslie's body was telling her that she wasn't eating right.

I suspected that Leslie's problems stemmed from food intolerance. She had been eating a high-FI diet for years, including all the supposedly healthy choices: eggs, tofu, whole-grain bread, whey protein shakes. She lived on diet sodas and café lattes with skim milk. Sometimes she'd treat herself to some corn chips and salsa. That made at least 6 of the 7 high-FI foods right there: eggs, soy, gluten, dairy, artificial sweeteners and corn. All she was missing was sugar and peanuts, and when she occasionally ate desserts or processed foods (which are often made with peanut oil), she was consuming those, too.

"Look," I told Leslie, as gently as I could, "you can be doing all the right things—exercise, careful eating, the works—but if you've built up a food intolerance or messed up your digestive tract, even the right things can't help you. Right now, your immune system is on high alert, and it's overreacting to many of the foods you eat. Until we get your immune system to chill out, you won't be able to lose weight."

Food intolerance is one of the most frustrating conditions I know. All of a sudden, you can't lose those extra pounds, even when you are eating and exercising exactly as you always have. Sometimes you might even be eating less and exercising more—and you still gain weight! How unfair is that?

The best way to get Leslie's immune system back on track was to cut out all 7 high-FI foods and increase her intake of low-FI foods. Once her immune system wasn't jumping into hyperalert and flooding her system with inflammatory chemicals, her digestive system would have a chance to heal. I also suggested my special Virgin Diet Shakes as a source of protein. Along with the healing foods and healing supplements I recommend, the Virgin Diet Shakes would help reverse inflammation, reducing all those "protective" chemicals that were causing Leslie's body to gain weight, aging her skin and hair and sapping her energy. In 7 days, I promised Leslie she would lose the bloat and look years younger. The Virgin Diet was the key.

In fact, that's exactly what happened. When I saw Leslie a few weeks later, she was so excited that her words kept tumbling over each other. "I've lost more than 10 pounds already, and I feel so hopeful about the other 30! Look at my skin. It hasn't looked this good in years! My friends keep asking if I was away on vacation. At work, they know I wasn't, so they've started a rumor about me having a new boyfriend. I can't believe how good I feel!"

I was so happy for my client because she had finally stopped accepting the weight gain, exhaustion and premature aging that she had come to believe was her lot in life. Instead, she was losing weight, feeling great and looking 10 years younger. Terrific was now her new normal. It can also be yours.

## STOP COUNTING CALORIES

So, what's the first thing I'd like you to do on the Virgin Diet? I hope you're sitting down because my first piece of advice might shock you: *stop counting calories.*

That's right, I'm suggesting that you stop counting calories because your body is not a savings bank or a calorimeter. It's a chemistry lab. Although the total number of calories counts, it is only part of the story. The *source* of the calories matters far more. If your calories come from foods that are causing your body trouble, then it almost doesn't

> Your body is not a savings bank or a calorimeter. It's a chemistry lab.

matter how much or how little you eat. Even moderate intake of problem foods sets up your body for weight gain. And as we've seen, those problem foods are not just cookies, cake and full-sugar soda. They include artificial sweeteners and diet sodas, low-fat yogurt, eggs, soy and whole grains.

 ## NO MORE MODERATION

Now here's the key to the Virgin Diet: when it comes to weight loss and healthy eating, *moderation doesn't work.*

Why? Because weight gain among the nonobese is generally gradual, averaging almost a pound a year as the result of only moderate changes in diet and activity. Yes, if you binge for months on potato chips and

> **Moderation doesn't work.**

ice cream, you're going to put on weight quickly. But that's not how most people gain weight. They continue eating their normal diet, with maybe just a tablespoon of butter here or a few extra cookies there. Before they know it, they've gained a pound a year, which adds up to 10 pounds in 10 years and 20 pounds in 20 years. It looks like age itself is the problem, but it's not. It's that pound a year that caused all the trouble.

In other words, the average 30-year-old who consumes a moderate caloric diet while eating the wrong foods will be 10 pounds heavier by age 40 for what may seem like no reason at all. And if at any point along the way that person tries to lose weight—usually by restricting calories—she's going to find it very difficult to lose weight, keep it off or both.

Why? Because, you guessed it, your body is not a bank account or a calorimeter. It is a chemistry lab. Eating the wrong foods affects your body's chemistry. Gaining weight affects your body's chemistry. Stress and lifestyle changes affect your body's chemistry. So, if you want to get that extra weight off, you have to *heal* your body's chemistry.

## QUIZ: WHAT ARE YOU TOLERATING?

Are you still not sure whether food intolerance is the cause of your weight gain and premature aging? Take this quiz and find out.

### IS FOOD INTOLERANCE HOLDING YOU HOSTAGE?

- If you have one of the symptoms listed below 1 to 2 times a week at a mild or moderate level—even if you barely notice it—score 2 points.
- If you have mild or moderate symptoms 3 or more times a week or a severe symptom 2 or more times a week, score 4 points.

| | | | |
|---|---|---|---|
| ____ | Abdominal cramping | ____ | Eczema |
| ____ | Acne/rosacea | ____ | Fatigue |
| ____ | ADD and Hyperactivity | ____ | Food cravings |
| ____ | Arthritis (osteo or rheumatoid) | ____ | Gas and bloating |
| | | ____ | Headaches |
| ____ | Asthma | ____ | Inability to lose weight |
| ____ | Brain fog | ____ | Joint pain |
| ____ | Chronic mucus/stuffy nose | ____ | Moodiness |
| ____ | Congestion | ____ | Muscle pain |
| ____ | Constipation and/or diarrhea | ____ | Psoriasis |
| | | ____ | Sinusitis |
| ____ | Dark circles under the eyes | ____ | Skin rashes |
| ____ | Depression | ____ | Throat clearing |

**TOTAL POINTS:** _____

**Your Food Intolerance Score:**

### 1 to 5: Low-FI

Currently, you seem to suffer from few food allergies or intolerances, if any. I have found that most people feel and look better while removing high-FI foods and often are reacting to one or more of them whether or not they have any overt symptoms. You are reading this book because you want to make sure that you eat the best diet so you can keep feeling and looking lean and young.

### 6 to 14: Mid-FI

You consistently suffer mild or moderate discomfort and bloating with certain foods, but you do experience periods of relief. Over time, you have probably noticed weight gain even though your diet hasn't changed. Your skin and hair may look somewhat dull, and you tend to feel more tired or stressed than you used to.

### 15+: High FI

Help! You can't remember the last time you felt light and lean after a meal, and it feels as though your stomach is constantly bloated. You've done everything you can think of to lose weight, and it just hasn't worked. Every time you look in the mirror, you think, *How did I get so old? Why do I look so tired?*

# FOOD IS INFORMATION

**Food isn't just calories or fat grams or even a source of energy.**

Okay, so here's how I like to think of it: food isn't just calories or fat grams or even a source of energy, food is information. Each bite of food that you put into your mouth sends your body a message—maybe even several messages.

Some of these messages relate to your blood sugar and insulin production. Some of them govern your feelings of hunger and fullness. Others concern your fat burning and metabolism, and still others involve your hair, skin, mood and mental functioning.

This is why I say that not all calories are created equal. You might portion out a cookie, a hamburger and a serving of cauliflower so they all have the same number of calories, but each of those three foods is going to send your body very different messages. And it's the messages we care about, not just the calories.

Actually, it's not just *what* you eat that gives your body information. It's also *how much* you eat at one time, *how fast* you eat, *what combinations* you eat, *how you feel* while you are eating and even *what you drink* with what you eat. Every one of those things is important because each sends your body a message: burn fat or store it; build muscle or lose it; slow the aging process down or speed it up; create steady, sustained energy or crash and burn within the next couple hours. Don't worry if this sounds complicated: I have laid it all out for you. All you have to do is

> Not all calories are created equal.

live by the Virgin Diet Plate and follow my rules of meal timing, and you will be golden. The Virgin Diet is designed to send only the right messages to your body—24/7 for 21 days. I'm betting that you'll like the feeling so much that you'll keep sending all the right messages for a long, long time after that.

 ## FOOD ALLERGIES: RARE BUT DANGEROUS

Food allergies are actually rather rare, but they get all the bad press because they are responsible for the really dramatic food problems that we hear about, such as the child who takes one bite of a peanut and then has to be rushed to the hospital. Food allergies trigger special antibodies in the bloodstream known as immunoglobulin E, or IgE, the most aggressive defense system our bodies have. Among other chemicals, IgE antibodies release large amounts of *histamine*, a substance that causes swelling, mucus, congestion and all the other symptoms that you would normally modify with an *antihistamine*.

It's the swelling reaction that makes food allergies so dangerous. In severe cases, the throat and airways become so swollen that they cut off the air supply, making you unable to breathe.

Even without such deadly responses, however, aggressive IgE antibodies generally produce quick, dramatic reactions, appearing within minutes or even seconds after the offending food is consumed. Other allergic reactions include rashes, hives, itching, eczema, nausea, stomach pain, diarrhea, shortness of breath and chest pain, as well as bloating, nausea, cramping and stomachache. Because much of our immune system is located in the gut, food allergies tend to wreak havoc with digestion.

Now, at this point, you might be thinking, *But I don't have any of those symptoms, and I feel fine after I eat.* If that's your response, terrific! You probably don't have any food allergies. Most people don't. But most people do have food intolerance, so let's take a closer look at that.

 ## FOOD INTOLERANCE: COMMON AND PROBLEMATIC

*Food intolerance* is an umbrella term that covers three ways other than food allergies that things can go wrong: true intolerance, food sensitivities and food reactions.

# TRUE INTOLERANCE

Some people's bodies simply have trouble tolerating certain foods, such as gluten (found in many grains, pastas, baked goods and processed and prepared foods), lactose (found in dairy products) or MSG (monosodium glutamate, a form of salt used as a flavor enhancer in many processed and prepared foods). Usually, this is because the intolerant people are lacking a specific chemical or enzyme that they need to digest the food. This is simply a genetic problem, and there isn't much you can do about it except to avoid the foods. The good news is that on the Virgin Diet, you will avoid these difficult foods, which will make it easier for you to lose weight, look younger and feel healthier.

# FOOD SENSITIVITIES

Like allergies, food sensitivities are a type of immune reaction, but they mobilize a different type of antibody than food allergies do—not IgE, but its cousin, immunoglobulin G, or IgG. These IgG antibodies produce symptoms, too, but they act more slowly than IgE antibodies. Whereas allergic reactions are swift, food sensitivity symptoms don't appear until several hours or even a few days after you've eaten, making it very difficult to link them to the problem food.

> Food sensitivities keep your immune system fired up on a chronic basis.

Here's another way in which allergic responses differ from sensitive ones: allergic responses are acute, whereas sensitivity responses are chronic. In other words, an allergy is a specific response: your immune system is activated, it flares up, it sends out its aggressive battery of IgE antibodies, and hopefully, it calms down. Food sensitivities, by contrast, can keep your immune system fired up on a chronic basis because you keep consuming the foods that set them off. If yogurt, eggs, soy milk and whole-wheat bread are a frequent part of your diet—and especially if you're eating them every day—your system is overwhelmed with problem foods, and your immune system never really calms down. This creates a number of problems, particularly inflammation, as I'll explain a bit later. But first, let's play food detective. Here are the typical symptoms of food sensitivity. Do any of them sound familiar to you?

- Digestive trouble, such as bloating, gas, constipation or diarrhea
- Sleep issues, such as fatigue, insomnia or waking in the middle of the night
- Congestion, sneezing and coughing
- Muscle aches and joint pain
- Dark circles under your eyes
- Dull, lifeless hair
- Skin problems, including acne and rosacea
- Mood problems, such as lack of focus, brain fog, depression, anxiety or irritability
- Poor or unsteady energy
- Weight gain
- Premature aging

If you're struggling with any of these symptoms, you are almost certainly struggling with food sensitivities and perhaps with other types of food intolerance as well.

Food sensitivity is incredibly common. It affects at least 75 percent of us and is a major factor in weight gain and weight retention. Again, the good news is that the Virgin Diet will help you cope with your food sensitivities, first by pulling problem foods from your diet and then by healing your system so you might eventually be able to tolerate some of those foods.

## FOOD REACTIONS

When you load your body up with too many carbs or too much sugar, you're setting yourself up for blood sugar spikes and crashes. This in turn messes with your *insulin response*—your body's attempt to move sugar out of your blood and into your cells. Your insulin response works best when your blood sugar levels are nice and steady and in the ideal range. The Virgin Diet supports this process and helps you avoid food reactions by having you eat ideal amounts of clean, lean protein; healthy fats; nonstarchy veggies; and high-fiber, low-glycemic carbs every 4 to 6 hours. Yes, pulling the top 7 high-FI foods is important, but so is the timing of your meals and the combinations of foods you eat. Consuming something sweet or high-carb—a piece of cake, a handful of dried fruit or even a glass of orange juice—causes your blood sugar to spike and messes with your insulin response. As you'll see in Chapter 7, artificial sweeteners can also create adverse reactions. Anything that interferes with blood sugar and insulin response disrupts your stress hormones—all of which makes you more likely to gain and retain weight.

 ## INFLAMMATION: FANNING THE FLAMES

Food intolerance produces a host of symptoms, which is bad enough. But it also causes a number of interrelated problems, each of which makes all the others worse. One of those problems is *inflammation,* a major cause of weight gain and weight-loss resistance.

Ironically, inflammation is a necessary by-product of any intense immune response—that is, it's supposed to help your system heal. When your body is invaded by a toxin, bacteria or a virus or traumatized by a wound, your immune system swiftly triggers a cascade of healing and protective chemicals that rush to the site. You can think of your immune system as an ambulance that comes roaring to the rescue after an accident.

But suppose the ambulance driver is so anxious to reach you that he crashes right through the side of your house? That's inflammation—the negative side effects of the healing process.

> Inflammation puts on the pounds in a number of different ways.

The four classic inflammatory responses are redness, heat, pain and swelling, symptoms that are easily visible when the injury can be seen. Think of how a cut on your finger turns red and how warm and tender the skin becomes, or imagine how a bugbite on your ankle might swell. Those reactions occur inside your body, too, when a high-FI food triggers an immune reaction. Your digestive tract becomes inflamed. If you frequently eat foods that inflame your system—either foods to which you're sensitive or foods that contain inflammatory fats (e.g., dairy, eggs and corn)—then you're likely to suffer from chronic low-grade inflammation. And you're running the risk of weight-loss resistance and obesity.

Inflammation puts on the pounds in a number of different ways:

- **Chemical changes.** Inflammation makes your body resistant to key chemical messengers that help you burn fat, tolerate stress and normalize your appetite and cravings. For example, inflammation keeps your body from "hearing" cortisol, the key stress hormone. As a result, your cortisol levels rise, stressing you out, storing fat around your waist and causing you to crave carbs. Cortisol also lowers your serotonin, the feel-good brain chemical that helps you feel calm and optimistic and sleep well. Eventually, your body gets tired of producing all that excess cortisol, and your levels drop, causing you to feel sluggish, unmotivated and fatigued.

Inflammation also creates resistance to leptin, the hormone that regulates feelings of hunger and fullness. Leptin resistance means that leptin can't get into your cells. This makes you hungrier, so you eat more, well past the point where your brain would normally be signaling "enough."

Finally, inflammation keeps your body from responding properly to adiponectin, which helps regulate blood sugar and body fat. Add up all these responses, and you get weight gain.

- **Insulin resistance.** Insulin is a hormone that moves sugar out of your bloodstream and into your cells. When I say, "sugar," I don't just mean the sweet white stuff that sits on the table. I mean the starches found in grains, the fructose and glucose found in fruits and vegetables and the lactose found in milk. These sugars enter your blood, where they are meant to provide energy for your body and brain, as long as insulin helps move them into your cells.

> Insulin resistance slams the doors to your fat cells shut.

But when you are consuming too much sugar (in the form of sweets, starches or dairy products) or when your system is inflamed, your body secretes too much insulin and keeps the insulin in your bloodstream longer than it's supposed to. After a while, your cells can't "hear" all that excess insulin. Your insulin receptors stop responding to the insulin, and your blood sugar remains high. You may eventually have trouble manufacturing enough insulin, putting you at risk for diabetes. Meanwhile, you can't use that extra blood sugar for energy, and it ends up getting stored as fat.

In addition, all that excess insulin in your blood tells your body you have enough sugar around for fuel, so it doesn't need to burn stored fat. Insulin resistance basically slams the doors to your fat cells shut. Insulin resistance also makes it nearly impossible to lose weight. And inflammation virtually guarantees that you will suffer from insulin resistance.

- **Fluid retention.** Inflammation doesn't just help you hold onto your body fat, it also causes you to retain fluids so you feel bloated and heavy.

- **Digestive problems.** When inflammation rages through your intestines, your digestive system can't operate efficiently. If you have an imbalance of gut bacteria, with more bad bacteria than good, you will actually extract more calories from the food you eat and store them as fat. If your gut wall is damaged and leaky, you will struggle to be able to absorb your nutrients. The result is that even though you are eating, you still feel hungry and unsatisfied because your body can't get what it needs from your food.

- **Loss of energy.** Inflammation causes you to feel sluggish and fatigued. If your body is inflamed, you are not going to feel like moving much, so you become even more sedentary. The less active you are, the more resistant to insulin you become—and the vicious cycle continues.

I hope you're beginning to see why I told Leslie to pull out of her diet any high-FI foods that might be causing an inflammatory response. The fastest way to gain weight that you can't lose is to allow your body to become inflamed. And the fastest way to drop those extra pounds is to remove the sources of inflammation and let your body heal. That's what the Virgin Diet is all about.

## INFLAMMATION: A SERIOUS WARNING SIGN

If you want to know whether your body is inflamed, ask your physician to test your blood for high-sensitivity C-reactive protein (hs-CRP). Even a slightly elevated hs-CRP level is associated with obesity and weight gain—and even worse, it's a predictor of diabetes, heart attack and stroke. Luckily, the Virgin Diet can help you bring those levels down quickly.

## FAT MAKES MORE FAT

As we just saw, inflammation causes you to gain and retain weight in several different ways—and those extra fat cells don't just sit there, either. They release more inflammatory chemicals, creating the mother of all vicious cycles. Inflammation can lead to obesity. And fat—especially belly fat—releases inflammatory chemicals called *cytokines,* which are messengers that your body uses to start the inflammatory process. So your fat cells are

> **Fat releases inflammatory chemicals called *cytokines.***

producing more inflammatory messengers, and all that inflammation is making you gain more weight, and then your fat is basically making you *more* fat! How unfair is that?

So all that extra fat you might be carrying around is not benign, like a backpack. It's more like carrying a bomb in your backpack. It's why I want you to lose fat quickly and lower inflammation quickly by pulling the 7 high-FI foods from your diet.

Following the Virgin Diet will also help you overcome insulin resistance. As part of the program, you'll eat every 4 to 6 hours and stick to moderate portion sizes of clean, lean protein; healthy fats; high-fiber, low-glycemic carbs; and nonstarchy vegetables. (I go into more detail about the program in Chapter 8.) This is the fastest way I know to get your blood sugar levels balanced and your insulin working efficiently once more.

## HOW YOU CREATE INFLAMMATION

- Eating foods to which your body is sensitive, allergic or intolerant

- Eating sugar, artificial sweeteners and processed and high-glycemic carbohydrates

- Eating pro-inflammatory fats, such as those found in eggs, corn and dairy

- Eating trans and damaged fats

- Having abdominal fat

#  INFLAMMATION AND LEPTIN RESISTANCE

Inflammation doesn't only create insulin resistance. It also creates leptin resistance, which makes it even harder for you to lose weight.

Leptin is a hormone that responds to how much you've eaten and signals the brain that you've had enough (*satiety* is the technical term). Leptin also helps burn fat by cueing your metabolism to run faster when you have extra fat to burn and slowing down your metabolism when your body needs to hold onto fat. You can see how our ancestors might have needed this hormone to help adjust their metabolisms depending on whether food was plentiful or scarce.

When leptin is working well, you eat until you don't need any more food and then you stop. When your system is leptin-resistant, you have a lot of leptin circulating in your blood, but your brain can't "hear" it. You end up with too much leptin in your blood and not enough in your brain. That's the situation for the vast majority of overweight people. As a result, they experience increased hunger, food cravings and weight gain. Even though they're overweight, their bodies believe they're hungry and go into a state of fat storage.

> If you want to lose that extra weight, you have to heal the leptin resistance.

If you want to lose that extra weight, you have to heal the leptin resistance. Healing inflammation will go a long way toward getting your leptin working properly again. And pulling the high-FI foods is key.

Meanwhile, if you keep eating high-FI foods, you continue to feed the problem. You might think you are making healthy choices with your nonfat yogurt, omega-3–rich eggs and low-fat soy milk, but every bite of high-FI food is potentially triggering an immune response that could

> Any time
> you eat a
> problem food,
> you're setting
> yourself up for
> weight gain.

flood your body with inflammatory chemicals and start the whole cycle over again. So basically, any time you eat a problem food, you're setting yourself up for weight gain.

All of the top 7 high-FI foods are potential sources of inflammation, which is why it's so important to pull them from your diet. Once you do so, your inflammation will disappear, your symptoms will disappear—and those extra pounds will disappear, too.

##  WHEN GOOD DIGESTION GOES BAD

There is another factor that might be making you fat and old before your time: poor digestion. When digestion works well, it is a beautiful thing, but when it's out of whack, it can be a huge contributor to weight gain.

Bacteria, also known as flora or gut flora, is crucial to good digestion. Believe it or not, we have more than 500 species of different bacteria in our gastrointestinal tract. In fact, we have more bacteria than we have cells. Most of that bacteria is good for us; it helps break down food, absorb nutrients and keep our immune systems primed. Some of that bacteria is bad—the kind that attacks our cells or produces toxins.

The key thing with gut bacteria is making sure that we have the ideal amount of good bacteria that we need. So, focus on promoting the good bacteria that will help support your gut immune system and keep the bad bacteria at bay.

How do you do that? First, protect your good bacteria. You might want to take *probiotics,* which are supplements that support bacterial growth. If you take antibiotics, which kill a lot of good bacteria while

# HOW TO REDUCE INFLAMMATION

- **Make an oil change.** Instead of consuming inflammatory fats from processed foods, corn, dairy and eggs, switch to anti-inflammatory fats from wild fish, raw nuts and seeds and olive oil. And make sure to avoid *damaged fats:* any oil that is rancid, refined or hydrogenated (trans fats). Damaged fats change the structure of your cell walls and make you more resistant to the messages from your hormones, including insulin and leptin, setting you up to put on weight and keep it on.

- **Get rid of the sugar, artificial sweeteners and high-glycemic foods.** There's a good reason sugar is on your top 7 high-FI list: sweet and starchy foods raise blood sugar, which raises insulin, which leads to inflammation. We'll learn more about high-glycemic foods in Chapter 7, and we'll also find out why artificial sweeteners are so bad for you—and your weight.

- **No more GMOs!** *Genetically modified organisms* (GMOs) are wrong in so many ways. They can disrupt your healthy *gut flora* (intestinal bacteria), trigger an immune response and create inflammation. The vast majority of soy and corn available in the United States is genetically modified, as we'll learn in Chapters 4 and 6.

- **Let go of the top 7 high-FI foods.** The top 7 high-FI foods are the ones most likely to cause an adverse reaction. Some, like dairy, gluten, soy, eggs, peanuts and corn, can trigger an immune response that leads to inflammation. Others, like sugar and artificial sweeteners, wreak havoc with your blood sugar. Either way, inflammation is the result.

they're gunning for the bad, upgrade probiotics from "good idea" to "absolutely essential." You always want to follow any antibiotic treatment with a round of probiotics.

You can further support your good bacteria with *prebiotics*, which is soluble fiber that feeds your gut flora (for example, garlic, onions, asparagus and dandelion greens), and with fermented foods, such as pickled ginger, kimchee and sauerkraut. We also need good gut bacteria to make vitamin K, which is important for immune function.

## THE ENEMIES OF GOOD DIGESTION

- Speed eating
- Drinking excess fluids with meals
- Eating when stressed
- Environmental toxins
- Antibiotics
- Pain medications
- Birth control pills
- Antacids (Yes, antacids! They lower the stomach acid you need to digest food.)
- Foreign travel
- High-FI foods
- A high-sugar diet
- Artificial sweeteners, colorings and flavorings
- Stress

## HEALTHY GUT, HEALTHY BODY

There is yet another piece to the inflammation–immune system puzzle: eating high-FI foods can contribute to a condition known as *leaky gut syndrome*.

Leaky gut is pretty much what it sounds like. The cells of your intestinal lining (your gut) are supposed to be pressed up tightly against one another, creating tight junctions. These junctions keep partially digested food securely inside your intestines, where it belongs.

Sometimes, though, your intestinal lining is compromised, allowing particles of partly digested food to leak out into your bloodstream. Other problematic stuff can get out, too, including microbes, waste and toxins.

When these substances enter your bloodstream, your body treats them as foreign invaders and responds accordingly. Your immune system releases a cascade of inflammatory chemicals designed to neutralize the threat, which can also wreak havoc on your intestinal lining. As a result, you have a much harder time absorbing nutrients, which might even cause you to eat more—and gain weight.

Eventually, the poorly digested food combines with IgG antibodies to form large bodies known as immune complexes. These circulate through the bloodstream until they are deposited in various tissues, where they create localized inflammation. That's how you end up with the symptoms we've talked about—the rashes, joint pain, headache, fatigue and skin eruptions.

All of these symptoms together can make you feel as though your whole body is breaking down. You might be tempted to think that this is what happens naturally as you age. It isn't. It's what happens when you suffer from leaky gut. If you've been eating the wrong foods for years, you'll probably develop more symptoms over time, as the problem worsens and symptoms build up.

Ironically, your body starts to crave the very foods that are making you sick. That's because if you keep eating high-FI foods, your body keeps making antibodies to protect you from them. If you try to cut out a particular high-FI food, you have all these antibodies roaming around in search of it, ready to zap it with their special protective chemicals. These would-be protectors actually cause you to crave the food they're longing to zap, setting you up for a vicious cycle of inflammation and weight gain.

Food intolerance can create leaky gut, but other factors can, too:

- Chronic inflammation
- Lactose intolerance
- Gluten as it triggers the release of the protein zonulin, which loosens the tight junctions in the gut
- A low-fiber, high sugar diet, which lowers your levels of stomach acid and contributes to leaky gut
- Poorly digested food, which may be caused by speed eating or stress eating
- A compromised immune system or an autoimmune condition, such as asthma, allergies or rheumatoid arthritis
- Overuse of nonsteroidal anti-inflammatory drugs (NSAIDS), such as aspirin and ibuprophen
- Infections, including viral, bacterial, yeast and parasitic
- Antibiotics
- Accutane (a form of vitamin A used to treat acne)
- Acid blockers
- Excessive alcohol consumption
- Cytotoxic drugs and radiation
- Exposure to heavy metals
- Exposure to molds

- Exposure to toxins
- GMOs, including such genetically modified foods as soy and corn, each of which averages about 90 percent of the U.S. crop

If you suffer from irritable bowel syndrome or irritable bowel disorder, you almost certainly have leaky gut as well.

The major cause of leaky gut, however—and the one that's been most challenging for me personally—is stress because it causes your gut to become more permeable. So if you've been going through an especially tough time or if your life is chronically stressful, those extra pounds (and unpleasant symptoms) might well be caused by both leaky gut and inflammation.

Leaky gut isn't just caused by food intolerance, it also *causes* food intolerance. As undigested food leaks through those open spaces in your gut, it makes its way into your bloodstream, and your immune system goes wild. Eventually, even foods that you were not previously sensitive to can become problem foods for you. So, we're looking at a vicious cycle in which leaky gut, inflammation and food intolerance all reinforce one another.

Here's the good news: if you remove the offending foods, your symptoms usually vanish, and the excess weight starts to come off. Once you heal your leaky gut, you might even become able to tolerate foods to which you are now sensitive. And the *really* good news is that you can heal leaky gut and perhaps also overcome at least some of your food intolerance through the Virgin Diet. When you drop the top 7 high-FI foods and load up on healing foods, you give your body a fresh, healing start. Meanwhile, you'll drop up to 7 pounds in 7 days and look years younger. It's a win–win.

# MY TOP GUT-HEALING NUTRIENTS

Think you have leaky gut? Here are some of my favorite supplements and healing foods that you can try in addition to cutting out the 7 high-FI foods.

## Healing Supplements

- **Plant digestive enzymes,** to support good digestion and reduce allergenic compounds (take 1 or 2 with each meal)
- ***Saccharomyces boulardii,*** to rebalance gut flora, prevent candida (yeast) overgrowth and support healthy gut immune function (250 to 500 milligrams per day)
- **Berberine,** to balance gut flora and blood sugar (1,000 to 2,000 milligrams per day)
- **Aged garlic extract,** an anti-inflammatory, antiviral, antifungal and antimicrobial powerhouse (1 to 3 caps per day)
- **Glutamine,** to heal leaky gut (1 to 10 grams per day, depending on severity)
- **Ginger,** an antioxidant that reduces inflammation and supports gut healing (30 to 50 milligrams per day)
- **Quercetin,** a natural antihistamine and antioxidant (100 milligrams per day)

## Healing Foods

- **Coconut milk,** rich in yeast-killing caprylic acid
- **Aloe juice,** to raise secretory IgA

- **Freshly ground flaxseed meal,** which contains a gluey substance that soothes and heals the gut, as well as omega-3s to reduce inflammation
- **Apples,** which contain pectins to heal the gut
- **Cold-water fish,** to reduce inflammation
- **Fresh garlic,** to reduce inflammation and kill off bad bacteria
- **Red onions,** which are rich in quercetin
- **Oregano leaves,** which are antifungal

## SLOW AND STEADY LOSES THE WEIGHT

Much of the reason for our poor digestion is how we eat. We eat too fast. I tell people, "Be a slowpoke when you're eating." Put your fork down in between bites. You can improve your digestion by increasing your chewing. Chew more. If we eat with people who eat fast, we tend to pace ourselves with them, so eat with slow people.

Mindful eating is not just taking the time to chew. It is also being calm while you're eating. Take time for your meals. Focus on what you're eating and the company around you—and don't eat while you're doing something else that needs your focus, such as driving or working. Keep your mind on the food and the pleasure of sharing it. You'll enjoy it more—and you'll eat less.

## THE ACID CONNECTION

Heartburn may be a sign that you're not producing enough stomach acid, which can happen when you're stressed out or agitated. It sounds paradoxical, but when you don't have adequate stomach acid to break down your food, food sits in your stomach longer than it should, and the acids keep washing up against your esophagus—which could be the cause of your heartburn.

If you experience heartburn *and* have a history of ulcers, talk to your doctor. Otherwise, try taking a good, comprehensive enzyme that contains betaine hydrochloride (HCL) and see how you feel. If your heartburn dissipates, you have the answer.

## POOPS YOU CAN BE PROUD OF

I don't want to gross you out, but now we need to talk about poops because they are a crucial part of digestion. Either diarrhea or constipation can indicate that you have problems digesting your food, which could ultimately affect your ability to lose weight.

Many people don't realize that they are suffering from constipation. When I say, "constipation," I want you to think three things:

1. **You're moving your bowels less than once a day.** Ideally, you should be going twice a day.

2. **You're having to really struggle.** Ideally, everything should come out nice and smooth.

3. **You're producing poops that are tiny or don't easily come all the way out.** That is not good for your digestive tract or your overall health.

What is a poop you can be proud of? It is a well-formed poop that you don't have to struggle with. It comes out fully—it doesn't stop halfway through and leave you stuck. Nor does it dive-bomb to the bottom of the bowl. It *sinks* to the bottom of the bowl. It doesn't mark things up.

If you have an oily residue or slick slides, you are not absorbing your fat well. If you have rabbit pellets or you're straining, you don't have enough fiber. If you have floating poops, it could be from excessive gas, produced by an overgrowth of bad bacteria lurking in your intestines.

Now at this point, you might be wondering why I'm putting you through this kind of gross science lesson. The answer is, because if you don't eliminate properly, you'll be bloated and fat and setting yourself up for a permanent problem with both indigestion and obesity.

Okay, I'll get a little more gross and ask you to picture what would happen to a poop that just sat in the toilet for a few days. Ewww, right? Well, do you want that toxic mess sitting inside you? No, you don't, and that's why elimination is so important. If you aren't having poops you can be proud of, you are holding a toxic mess inside your body every single day. That uneliminated poop is releasing toxins that are reabsorbed into your body, leading to bad breath, hemorrhoids and acne, not to mention impaired digestion, inflammation and food intolerance. The net result is that you gain weight that you can't lose, and you feel sluggish, tired and old before your time.

Those toxins are also putting a terrific strain on one of your primary detoxification organs: your liver. If you tax your liver with excess toxins, you could impair its ability to do its other critical functions, such as metabolize fat, which will ultimately make it more difficult for you to lose weight.

Maybe this isn't the most pleasant topic, but it's an important one—and what we focus on, we can improve. So at this point, I'd like to invite you to take my poop quiz.

## JJ'S POOP QUIZ: SKIP IT AT YOUR PERIL!

Now, I know we don't talk about poop much, and most of the time, there are very good reasons for that! The problem is, we have a broad range of what people think is normal—and a lot of that "normal" is really unhealthy. So this quiz is designed to help you identify what is actually normal—I mean, fully healthy—and what is not.

Answer yes to any of these questions if you are experiencing this symptom on an ongoing basis: for 1 month or longer and at least 2 or 3 times a week.

| | |
|---|---|
| _____ | Do you average less than one bowel movement per day? |
| _____ | Do you have incomplete evacuation? |
| _____ | Do you strain? |
| _____ | Are your stools hard? |
| _____ | Do your stools smell? |
| _____ | Are your stools mucus-like, light colored or greasy? |
| _____ | Do you pass smelly gas? |
| _____ | Are your stools stringy? |
| _____ | Do your stools resemble pellets? |
| _____ | Do you feel gassy or bloated, or do you have abdominal discomfort? |

____     Do your stools float?

____     Do you have diarrhea or loose stools?

____     Do you have an urgent bowel movement immediately after eating?

Okay, so here's the deal: none of these symptoms are normal, and you shouldn't experience any of them regularly on a long-term basis. You might have symptoms that occur periodically because of stress, a transient parasite, bad food—some problem that your body handles and you recover from. But if you have any of these problems *chronically*, you need to address them. And you should be aware that the more questions you answered yes to, the more severe your issue is.

Now, here's the good news: quite often, removing high-FI foods and adding in healing and low-FI foods correct most if not all of the problems. Here's some more good news: the Improving Your Poops section can tell you how to fix any remaining problems.

## IMPROVING YOUR POOPS

Now that you see how important pooping is for getting rid of toxins, let's talk about things that can help you poop better.

First, make time for it. Everyone has a rhythm. You will find your best time of day. For most people, it is when they get up in the morning or about an hour after they wake up and move. Make sure you have time for that. You may also need to have another bowel movement in the afternoon after lunch. Start to get used to what your body needs so you can set time aside. You need the right place to be able to do this, too.

Second, you need to have one to three bowel movements a day. They shouldn't be urgent, and you shouldn't have to run to the bathroom every time you eat. When you eat, it should stimulate some peristalsis in 30–60 minutes. (Peristalsis is the contraction and relaxation of your intestinal muscles to move food through your digestive tract.) But you should not be feeling the urgent need to run to the bathroom as soon as you finish your meal. If you pull all of the top 7 high-FI foods from your diet and your urgency hasn't cleared up in a couple weeks, see your doctor.

## Fiber

Fiber definitely gives us poops we can be proud of! You need fiber to add the bulk to your stools. Here are the top 10 sources of fabulous fiber, so load up on these:

1. Raspberries (All berries are high-fiber, and these are the highest.)
2. Lentils
3. Nuts
4. Seeds, especially chia seeds and freshly ground flaxseeds
5. Kale
6. Quinoa
7. Avocado
8. Apples
9. Winter squash
10. Broccoli

You need to eat optimal amounts of fiber. The average person is getting only 5 to 14 grams of fiber per day, but I want you to get it up to 50 or more. You can't do it overnight. Add 5 grams each day until you reach your goal—and make sure to drink more water as you do so.

## Water

In Chapter 8, you'll find my instructions for drinking water. Water and fiber together make a nice sponge that will give you the bulk you need in your stools.

## Supplements

- **Vitamin C:** Start with 1 gram and increase as needed up to 5 grams each night.
- **Magnesium:** Start with 300 milligrams and increase as needed up to 1,000 milligrams each night.

If your poops become runny, back off the supplements a bit. Iron and calcium are constipating, so if you are taking either of these, you may need some supplements to offset those effects. I like to take vitamin C and magnesium at night to get things moving in the morning.

## And Some Other Things...

- Get things moving with exercise.
- Try drinking some hot coffee or tea in the morning.
- Sip some peppermint tea throughout the day.
- Throw two or three prunes into your shake.
- When you move your bowels, consider elevating your feet with a footstool—our toilets are just about the worst possible setup for elimination.

If none of this is working, try cascara sagrada, senna, Chinese rhubarb and/or frangula (I prefer to use herbal blends of these) on a short-term basis. These are also great to take along if you happen to get constipated while traveling. You should only use them for a few days—don't become dependent on them, as they may irritate the gastrointestinal lining long term with chronic use.

# THE VIRGIN DIET: YOUR KEY TO WEIGHT LOSS

I know it's hard to believe that the foods you've always thought were healthy are actually causing you to gain weight, feel lousy and look at least 10 years older. But trust me, I've had thousands of clients—from students to CEOs to top Hollywood stars—lose stubborn extra pounds, look 10 years younger and feel better than they had in years. The Virgin Diet is the key for me, for them and for you.

> I've had thousands of clients lose extra pounds, look 10 years younger and feel better than they had in years.

If you're feeling skeptical, leaf through this book, read some of my clients' testimonials and see whether you recognize yourself in them. Most important of all, give the Virgin Diet a try. I'm only asking you for 21 days, and in return, I'm offering you a lifetime of feeling and looking your best.

Now, at this point, I'm going to give you a choice. If you're totally on board with my reasoning and just want to get to the weight loss, jump right on over to Chapter 2 for a full explanation of what you're going to be doing for the next 21 days and then turn to Part III to begin the Virgin Diet.

But if, like me, you don't like simply following orders and prefer to understand how your body works, read on. In the next chapter, you'll learn exactly how the Virgin Diet will help heal your body, and in

Part II, you'll find out just how the 7 high-FI foods are affecting your weight, your energy and your overall health. In other words, I'm going to give you the most useful chemistry lesson you've ever had in your life. This is the chemistry lesson that's finally going to help you understand why you haven't been able to lose weight before—and why you're finally going to be able to lose it now.

# HOW THE VIRGIN DIET WORKED FOR ME

**Karen Bristing**
**Age 48**

La Canada-
Flintridge,
California

**Height:**
5'7"

**Starting Weight:**
157 pounds

**Waist:** 31"
**Hips:** 41"

**Current Weight:**
142 pounds

**Waist:** 29.5"
**Hips:** 39.5"

**Lost:** 15 pounds

I first heard about JJ Virgin through her book *Six Weeks to Sleeveless and Sexy: The 5-Step Plan to Sleek, Strong, and Sculpted Arms.* I started implementing her program immediately—and seeing results—then I signed up for her online newsletter and heard about the concept of the Virgin Diet.

I had never tried eliminating gluten and dairy from my diet, never mind soy, corn, peanuts and eggs. I had been trying to lose a stubborn 5 pounds for years, but I was never able to do it on the traditional "eat less and exercise more" programs. And believe me, I tried them all! I had even tried extreme exercise, getting up at 5 a.m. for a grueling hour of outdoor boot camp. I did that for years!

I also fell prey to "diet" foods that were full of chemicals and artificial sweeteners. I was working out and I thought I was eating right. But the stress on my body kept me from ever getting below that number I hoped to see on the scale.

Now, I am working out less, eating according to JJ and loving it. I weigh less than I have in 10 years. Not only did I lose the elusive 5 pounds, but also another 10 fell off my body for a total of 15 pounds down! My skin is clearer, too. I found that as soon as I tried to add dairy back into my diet, my skin broke out. So dairy has stayed out of my life.

The great thing is, I really don't miss any of those foods. I have much more energy. My breakfast shake keeps me full until lunchtime. I no longer need to have some sugar after lunch to keep me going, and I don't feel the need for an afternoon nap anymore. I fit into all the clothes in my closet, although buying more jeans in a smaller size has been fun.

I am just so glad that I found this program. I've recommended it to my friends, and I enjoy seeing their successes as well. All I can say is that it has changed my life.

# HOW THE VIRGIN DIET

## CAN WORK FOR YOU

Jenna was a market analyst who routinely worked 12-hour days and rarely took a full day off. She was in her mid-30s, and she was as compulsive about her workout schedule as she was about her diet. She never took a bite she didn't plan, and she insisted on eating healthy, organic and lean foods. In fact, I would have to say that despite her demanding schedule, Jenna put about as much energy into staying healthy and fit as anybody I've ever seen.

Yet, for the past few years, Jenna had been struggling with slow but steady weight gain that didn't seem to respond to her efforts to step up her workouts or cut back on her occasional treats. By the time I started working with her, she was 30 pounds over her ideal weight—and just about frantic with frustration.

That was nothing, though, to how she reacted when I told her she would have to cut the 7 high-FI foods out of her diet. She didn't mind losing the sugar because she had pretty much cut it out anyway, and she was fine with giving up peanuts and corn, which she rarely ate. She could even wrap her mind around cutting out yeast and gluten because she was pretty much avoiding bread, pasta and baked goods already. But when she thought about cutting out her soy-laden protein bars, her low-fat Greek yogurt, her fresh-squeezed juice and her veggie omelets, I thought she was going to go ballistic. And when

I told her that diet sodas were off-limits, she was literally speechless for 2 minutes.

When she could finally speak, she said just four words: "JJ, are you *sure?*"

"I am."

Then she started to bargain with me. "Maybe I could have, like, *one* protein bar during the day? I don't think they have *much* soy—and I really need a high-protein snack I can eat at my desk. And maybe if I'm really good about the other things, I could have yogurt, like, *twice* a week? Or maybe *three* times? Ever since I gained all this weight, yogurt and berries are just about the only dessert I ever get—and the berries are healthy, right? And maybe as a special treat, I could have, say, *one* omelet on the weekend, if I don't use any butter and fry it in a nonstick pan? One omelet—that's only *two* eggs a week. I won't even use the yolks, just the whites! That's reasonable, right? I mean, moderation in all things, don't you agree?"

"Look," I told Jenna, "I know it's tough to cut out so much, and after 21 days you might be able to add some of these foods, like eggs or dairy, back into your diet. But if you want this diet to work, it's got to be 100 percent compliance for the next 21 days. You have to cut out every single one of the top 7 high-FI foods. I'm not talking 99 percent, I'm talking 100 percent."

"But why?" Jenna asked, almost in tears. For a minute, she sounded more like a distressed little girl than the high-powered financial wizard I knew she was.

I explained to Jenna that if she *wasn't* struggling with food intolerance, she would certainly have been able to lose her excess weight by now. So I had to assume that she was plagued with leaky gut, inflammation and digestive difficulties and that even small amounts of high-FI foods would make them worse. Jenna's gastrointestinal tract and her immune system were not functioning properly, and her stubborn weight gain was the result. To heal her body, we had to heal her leaky gut, cool her inflammation and give her immune system a chance to calm down. Even a single bite of egg or a spoonful of yogurt might be enough to undo all of her efforts.

Jenna reluctantly agreed to follow the Virgin Diet, and for the first 3 or 4 days, it was tough going. Her immune system was used to making antibodies that would zap the dairy, eggs and soy in her system, and now those antibodies were causing her to crave those foods intensely. For those few days, even though she was doing everything right, Jenna actually felt worse.

"Hang in there," I told her when she called me in despair. "This reaction is a *good* sign. You wouldn't be having such a hard time giving up these foods if you weren't sensitive to them. It's like with an addict; you know how serious the addiction is based on how tough the withdrawal symptoms are. Your cravings are telling us that we are totally on the right track, so just give it a few more days."

By the end of week 1, Jenna had started to feel better—especially when she realized that she had lost 7 pounds. By the end of week 2, she surprised herself with how clearheaded and focused she felt. By the end of week 3, she was thrilled to discover that she had lost a total of 10 pounds—and looked younger than she had in years.

Drop the top 7 high-FI foods for 21 days, lose up to 10 pounds or perhaps even more and look 10 years younger. It's easier than it sounds. And the results are soooo worth it.

# THE VIRGIN DIET: AN OVERVIEW

## Cycle 1: 21 days

- **Cut out** all of the top 7 high-FI foods.
- **Fuel your system** with healing foods and healing supplements.

## Cycle 2: 28 days

- **Every week for 4 weeks,** test one potentially healthy high-FI food: gluten, soy, eggs or dairy. Based on your responses, determine whether each food should stay or go.

## Cycle 3: Lifetime

- **Get moving:** incorporate the most effective exercise routine.
- **Avoid** corn, peanuts and sugar and artificial sweeteners 95 percent of the time.
- **Rechallenge** the potentially healthy high-FI foods that you reacted to in Cycle 2 after 3 to 6 months to see if you can now tolerate them.
- **Every 12 months,** repeat the program.

# HOW THE VIRGIN DIET WORKS

The Virgin Diet is a 3-cycle plan. In the first cycle, you cut out all of the top 7 high-FI foods. In the second cycle, you rechallenge your system each week with one of the four most reactive high-FI foods: soy, dairy, eggs or gluten. You might be able to tolerate some or all of these once your system has had a chance to heal, or you might have to let them go, at least for now. Finally, for the third cycle, I'll show you how to experience these benefits for life. Maintaining your weight and losing weight require different strategies, and I'll set you up to maintain your healthy diet while you also incorporate the exercise routine and lifestyle habits that are most effective for long-term success. You'll learn how to periodically check in with your body for food intolerances and why it's important for your health to eliminate the top 7 high-FI foods once a year.

If, like Jenna, you're feeling a bit overwhelmed, that's a natural reaction. Don't worry—it's much easier than it sounds. Although you might be in for a tough few days, you'll lose the cravings completely in 3 days. And you're going to feel terrific after your system gets rid of the food that has been making you fat, tired and old before your time. It's easier to stay motivated if you understand where you're going and why, so let me talk you through all three cycles of the Virgin Diet.

## CYCLE 1: ELIMINATION

The great thing about Cycle 1 is that you get to lose weight *fast*. This isn't a trivial thing. A recent study from the *International Journal of Behavioral Medicine* showed that people who lose weight fast are 5 times more likely to keep it off for 18 months than people who lose weight more slowly. To quote the study, "findings indicate both short- and long-term advantages to fast initial weight loss. Fast weight losers obtained greater weight reduction and long-term maintenance, and were *not* more susceptible to weight regain than gradual weight losers."[1]

One reason I have you cut out all of the top 7 high-FI foods is that I want you to lose weight quickly, and the best way to do that is to pull from your system everything that is potentially causing inflammation and messing with your blood sugar. You have to pull these foods out completely for a 3-week period to get rid of the immune complexes and IgG antibodies that are hanging around. When you pull the foods out, it will give your body a chance to recover from the inflammation and get rid of the immune complexes that are causing you uncomfortable symptoms such as joint pain, headaches, bloating, gas, fatigue and brain fog.

Eventually, the IgG antibodies will begin to dissipate. If you eat even a little bit of one high-FI food during this period, you will trigger the release of these IgG antibodies and create more immune complexes, thus unraveling your healing process.

I liken it to sitting on a chair on four tacks. You think, *This is hurting my butt.* You get up. You pull the tacks out but leave one tack behind. You sit back down. Your butt still hurts. It's the same thing with food intolerance and inflammation. Even one tack in your butt causes pain. Even one bite of a high-FI food keeps that inflammatory cycle going.

**Even one bite of a high-FI food keeps that inflammatory cycle going.**

As you pull out the high-FI foods, you'll learn which foods you should add into your diet and the best ways to eat them to maintain steady blood sugar and improve digestion. I'm going to tell you why clean, lean protein is good for you and can tame your appetite and cravings. I'm going to explain why berries and apples are healthy. I'm going to prod you to eat your green leafies—kale, collards, chard—along with healthy vegetables like broccoli and cauliflower.

But I'm also going to help you become mindful of how much you're eating and when. *Too much healthy food isn't healthy.* You'll learn how to eat the right amounts at the right times so your body can heal and drop fat fast. I promise that after those first 3 days, you'll get rid of the cravings, and you won't feel hungry.

## CYCLE 2: REINTRODUCTION

I've always had trouble with "one size fits all" approach programs for anything. We are all so different. So in Cycle 2, we'll customize your diet and discover which high-FI foods are really causing *you* trouble. In this cycle, I will show you how to safely test four of the high-FI foods—gluten, soy, dairy and eggs—to see if you can incorporate them back into your diet.

You might be wondering how you'll know if you are intolerant to one of these foods. After all, you may have been eating them for years, possibly every day, without noticing a problem. Trust me, you'll know! The beauty of this program is the science behind it. In Cycle 1, we lower your IgG load and get rid of the inflammation in your body. Once you have lowered your IgG load, you will feel even worse if you eat a food you're sensitive to than you did before. You will have more profound symptoms.

Once you know which foods cause reactions, you can tailor your diet to your personal body chemistry. I'll show you how to incorporate the right foods back into your diet in *healthy* ways. I'll explain when it's important to eat organic; how to tell safe, healthy eggs from unhealthy ones; and how much of these foods to eat on a regular basis.

The good news is that even if you can't handle one of these foods after 21 days, that won't necessarily be the case for life. Let's say that eggs cause you trouble (which they do initially for 70 percent of my clients). You might find that in another 3 to 6 months of healing your gut, you will be fine with them, so you can check back later and retest.

Will you ever put corn, peanuts, sugar or artificial sweeteners back in as mainstays of your diet? I hope not! As I explain in Part II, these foods tend to inflame you, aggravate your immune system and potentially drive up your blood sugar and insulin, so you want to avoid them at least 95 percent of the time.

But don't worry, you won't even miss them. In fact, most people get to the end of the 3 weeks and say that they don't want to try putting all the foods back into their diets. You will feel so much different by day 22 that you won't want to go back either. Trust me.

## CYCLE 3: THE VIRGIN DIET FOR LIFE

In Cycle 3, I give you some real specifics about what maintenance looks like. When you look at most weight-loss plans, their whole focus is on those first few weeks. They don't have any specifics on how to maintain your new weight. Not surprisingly, if you look at diet statistics, you see anywhere from a 50 percent to a 95 percent failure rate.

That's because the activities you need to do for successful maintenance are different from the activities that you need to do to be successful in fast weight loss. There was an interesting study in the *American Journal of Preventive Medicine* showing that of the 36 practices associated with successful weight loss, only 8 were associated with weight-loss maintenance. The study concluded that "Successful weight loss and weight-loss maintenance may require two different sets of practices."[2]

Okay, so the problem is that planning for maintenance is just not sexy. I get it. Maintenance isn't fun. What's fun is losing 7 pounds in 7 days. What's fun is dropping a bunch of dress sizes and getting all new clothes. But when your body is just the way you want it to be, and you *still* have to keep working, it just doesn't seem fair.

The key is to keep things exciting and come up with new rewards and incentives to maintain your new look. In Cycle 3, I'll teach you ways to help you remember how much you love your new healthy, slender body. I will show you how to keep the Virgin Diet fresh so you keep the weight off for good. I promise!

## MODERATION WILL MAKE YOU FAT

I'm sure you've heard this saying: "Everything in moderation." That drives me nuts! The truth is that moderation makes people overweight over time. It gives them license to eat things they shouldn't eat. As far as I'm concerned, moderation is the enemy.

> Moderation is the enemy.

If something is not good for you, is a little bit of it okay? Once you know something is not good for you, why would you want any exposure to it at all if you can control it? There is no safe level of trans fats, high-fructose corn syrup or artificial sweeteners. Avoid them completely not moderately.

Moderation makes you fat for several different reasons:

- **Moderation creates a slippery slope.** If a little bit is okay, then a little bit more is still okay. The next thing you know, that one cookie turns into two, and that weekly sugary muffin turns into a daily ritual.

- **Moderation sets you up for cravings.** If you don't eat chips, then you won't think about chips. The minute you eat chips, what do you think about? Eating more chips. That's one of the things

I hate about artificial sweeteners: when you eat sweet, you crave sweet. You have a little bit of something, and it makes you want more and more.

We are better off looking at an artificial sweetener and thinking, *This is toxic. This will hurt me.* The high-FI foods will hurt you, especially as they accumulate in your system. Plus, we all have trigger foods, and just a little bit of them creates desire. It doesn't take much to create weight gain.

- **Moderation sets you up for addiction to foods.** This is especially true with processed foods, which usually contain gluten, dairy or both. Gluten peptides and the casein peptides in dairy products can react with opiate receptors in the brain, thus mimicking the effects of opiate drugs like heroin and morphine.[3, 4] As a result, they can have a drug-like effect on the brain. Dr. Neal Barnard, author of *Breaking the Food Seduction: The Hidden Reasons Behind Food Cravings—and 7 Steps to End Them Naturally,* says:

  Cheese, for example, is loaded with casein, a protein that breaks up during digestion to produce morphine-like opiate compounds called casomorphins. These substances are thought to contribute to the mother–infant bond that occurs during nursing. A cup of milk contains about six grams of casein, and skim milk contains a little more, but casein becomes even more concentrated in the production of cheese. So it's no surprise that many of us feel bonded to our pizzas. Chocolate, sugar, and meat work in slightly different ways, but they all release drug-like substances that seduce the brain into coming back for more.[5]

In his book *The End of Overeating*, Dr. David Kessler likewise talks about how the sugar/salt/fat combination of most processed foods creates an addiction that makes it virtually impossible to eat these foods in moderation: "Until you have gained the upper hand over trigger foods, an attempt at moderation won't work."[6] In other words, if you have a little bit, you will want a little bit more and more.

- **Moderation allows immune complexes to accumulate.** Most of us get small amounts of toxins all day every day from food or from what we drink or breathe. No matter the source, what we can't get rid of will accumulate in our bodies.

  It's the same with food sensitivities. They produce immune complexes, and some of those complexes can accumulate. If you eat a little bit of a high-FI food each day, you are just building up more complexes. That "moderate" consumption over time can create chronic reactions from your gastrointestinal system and your immune system and ultimately impact your weight.

- **Moderation ignores the serious damage that foods can do.** If you're using the bank-account model, you might think, *Oh, it's just 100 extra calories each day. What harm could that do?* But your body is not a bank account, it's a chemistry lab. Food is not just food, it's also information. What message is it sending your body? What happens if you add a 100-calorie snack every afternoon to your diet, say, some crackers or a couple cookies?

> Food is not just food, it's also information.

You're not just consuming 100 calories. You're consuming gluten that can damage your gut, plus sugar that is raising your blood sugar and keeping insulin in your bloodstream. That extra insulin tells your body to store more fat. If the snack was made with any of the 7 high-FI foods—and virtually all processed foods have at least one of those ingredients—you have high-FI foods causing an inflammatory response, which then triggers insulin resistance (making it harder to lose weight), leptin resistance (keeping you hungry even when you've had enough) and cortisol resistance (making you feel either more stressed out, more fatigued or both). Then you get cravings from the immune complexes that start to form, and your blood sugar crashes way too soon. You don't have the right insulin or leptin response keeping you from feeling hungry, and now you want a second snack and a third and a fourth. I'd love to do a study that shows how many people actually stop with one 100-calorie snack.

The bottom line is that moderation is a big part of the problem. Moderation really is making you fat.

## SO WHAT CAN I EAT?

I've spent a lot of time telling you what not to eat, and most likely you are currently eating most if not all of these 7 foods every day. Almost 90 percent of what the average American eats is processed food, and that processed food usually contains corn, soy or both. Besides corn and soy, most processed foods contain gluten, dairy, eggs, peanuts, sugar or artificial sweeteners. When I tell people to pull these 7 high-FI foods, they ask, "What will I eat?" The truth is, eating and planning meals becomes very simple.

On the Virgin Diet, you may not have as many choices, but the ones you have are great. You eat chicken. You eat turkey. You eat wild fish. You eat grass-fed beef. You drink protein-rich Virgin Diet Shakes. Those are your lean proteins. You eat sweet potatoes, black beans, lentils, legumes, brown rice, quinoa, apples and berries. Those are your high-fiber, low-glycemic starchy carbs. You eat raw nuts and seeds, coconut, avocado, olive oil and palm fruit oil. Those are your healthy fats. You eat loads of nonstarchy vegetables. Without all those processed foods in your system, the subtle flavors of the vegetables and the natural sweetness of the berries start to taste delicious.

> You won't feel hungry. You won't feel deprived. You'll just feel better.

You don't need to spend big money to eat this way. When you don't buy boxes of crackers, cereal and frozen processed products, you may actually save money. With all the delicious, healthy food you'll be eating, you won't feel hungry. And with all the healthy alternatives to the high-FI foods, you won't feel deprived. You'll just feel better.

Now, you will need to be vigilant. Over the new few weeks, you will become mindful of exactly what is in your food. It will probably shock you to find out all the places where soy, gluten, dairy and eggs are hidden. You will be astonished to realize how many things are sweetened with sugar or artificial sweeteners. You will be amazed to realize how often peanuts lurk in our food—even in a "healthy" protein bar.

> We were never meant to eat the same thing all day every day.

You will think, *Oh my gosh. Who knew that I was eating this stuff all day every day?* We were never meant to eat the same thing all day every day. We were also not meant to have soy and corn in everything we eat.

#  KEEPING IT SIMPLE

One of the important things about the Virgin Diet is to help you avoid eating the same highly reactive foods all the time. So, you're going to rotate your proteins and enjoy a variety of nonstarchy vegetables. However, too much variety and choice can create problems as well—just think *buffet* to understand why.

To keep it simple and easy, you will have my Virgin Diet Plate to use as your guideline. You will always have clean, lean proteins, such as wild-caught fish or organic chicken. You will eat some high-fiber, slow-release carbs. You will eat healthy fats to reduce inflammation. You will eat loads of nonstarchy vegetables.

Once you fall into the pattern, it will be easy for you to stick to the plan. That's why in Chapter 11, instead of a meal plan, which would tell you exactly what to eat each day, I give you The Ultimate Meal Assembly Guide for you to learn how to put together proteins, high-fiber carbs, fats and nonstarchy vegetables into satisfying and healthy combinations. I give you a few key options: the stoup (a cross between stew and soup), the bowl, the salad, the wrap and the plate. I give you lists of healthy foods and show you how to pick the right amounts from each list—and the rest is up to you.

Once you learn how to assemble meals, you will find that eating according to the Virgin Diet is just as easy as the way you eat now. Maybe even easier. And it will almost certainly be less expensive because you won't be wasting money on processed foods.

# KEEPING A FOOD JOURNAL

In addition to tracking your progress, I also want you to keep a food journal throughout Cycles 1 and 2: a record of what you eat and how you feel every single day. After Cycle 2, you can let it go—unless you feel yourself starting to slip. Tracking is one of the best ways to keep yourself on track. In fact, I think journaling is such an essential part of your success that I "fire" clients who won't do it. Don't make me fire you, too!

Why do I want you to keep a food journal? Here are just some of the benefits:

- **You can identify what triggers a problem.** Throughout this book, I'm going to tell you every place that high-FI foods hide, but something might sneak in that you didn't even know you ate. All of a sudden—especially if this happens at the end of week 2 or during week 3—you feel rotten again. Then you will think, *What the heck did I do that's laying me out?* Remember, food intolerance is sneaky; it might take a few days to show up. If you have tracked every bite in your food journal, then you'll be much more likely to identify the culprit—and you will have learned something very important about which foods cause you problems.

- **What you measure, you can improve.** That's why I want you to write everything down. I have to laugh when people just write down the good days. No! You must write it *all* down.

- **You can easily forget how much progress you've made.** I definitely want you to track your symptoms and then look back and say, "Wow." Otherwise, you get through 3 weeks and say,

"I wasn't feeling that bad." If you read back through your journal and remember it all—the headaches, the mood swings, the acne, the fatigue—you realize that your old normal and your new normal are miles apart. That gives you motivation to lose the rest of your weight, if you haven't yet hit your ideal, and it keeps you inspired to make the most of your maintenance plan so this new terrific normal stays that way.

And don't just take my word for it! Jack Hollis, PhD, is one of the researchers at Kaiser Permanente's Center for Health Research in Portland, Oregon, on one of the largest and longest-running weight-loss maintenance trials ever conducted. The trial has shown that the more food records people kept, the more weight they lost. As Dr. Hollis reported, "Those who kept daily food records lost twice as much weight as those who kept no records. It seems that the simple act of writing down what you eat encourages people to consume fewer calories."[7]

Check out a sample journal page you can download from my website at www.thevirgindiet.com/journal.

 ## GET INSPIRED

This exercise is for those times when you need just a little bit more motivation. There will always be naysayers and doubters who may try to drag you down. You know who they are: the friends who tell you that weight gain is unavoidable, that your metabolism slows as you get older, that you shouldn't even dream of fitting into those jeans from high school.

Well, don't listen to them! Sure, if you are 5 feet tall with a larger frame, you won't ever be 6 foot tall and petite. That's not realistic. But you *can* be the best you've ever been in your life *at any point in your life* if you make the decision and focus on what you need to do to get there.

So let's get inspired. Let's set some goals that will stretch you and motivate you. You need goals that will get you excited enough to get off the couch and do what you need to do. You need to build a case for why you need to be doing this. What are the things that you want to have?

> Let's set some goals that will stretch you and motivate you.

Do you want to have great energy in the afternoon? Do you want to be able to wear a bikini at the beach and not feel self-conscious? Do you want to go to your high school reunion and feel like you're a rock star? Do you want to do sports with your kids? I take my kids to the gym, and they can't even keep up with me. Is that something you want in your life, too? Do you want to be able to zip up anything in your closet, have no cravings, get rid of headaches, never get sick and have great energy? What goals would make it worth it for you to totally take on the Virgin Diet?

Let's make a checklist. I want to know your top three goals for joining this program. Write them down. I want you to look at your checklist and see what success looks like for you. Is it being a size 8? Is it great energy? Is it no headaches? Is it to stop getting sick or stop having joint pain? Is it to lose the cravings?

Now I'd like you to make a list of your top three costs. What does it cost you if you *don't* do this program? Where are you right now? What's not working? Here's the reality: unless you make a change, your life is not going to get any better. You don't get better unless you do better. You don't get better if you don't change. Imagine if this is as good as it gets. What opportunities will you miss out on by not taking action? What are you sacrificing in terms of your career, your relationships, your happiness and your health?

You have to figure out what is most motivating to you. Some people are motivated by pleasure. Most people are more motivated by avoiding pain. It might be the pain of hurting all the time, not being able to think straight, being tired or not being able to do the things you really want to do because food is creating inflammation and getting in your way. Whatever your costs are, know that if you don't maintain the Virgin Diet, food will take you down.

Let's be clear. If you see it, you'll believe it. So, what would you look like if you were your ideal weight? There are great websites out there where you can actually scan in a picture and then see yourself looking thinner. (See the Resources section on my website.) Or find a photo of a body that you really like—your ideal body. Replace the person's head with your own via Photoshop or good old cut and paste. Make some copies of your new you. Put it in places where you need a little motivation and support. If you can see what you look like at your ideal weight, then you will start to live like a healthy, lean person. Think of that picture as your defender, your reminder and your support system.

Look, I know this program isn't easy. It's simple, but it isn't easy. There are going to be times when you feel like giving up. So, when you feel like you need motivation and inspiration, remember your top three goals. Why are you doing this? So you can have the relationship of your dreams and not feel self-conscious naked? So that you can play with your kids? What are those three things? Write them down and carry them around with you. Carry that picture, too. You need to see it to believe it.

> If you follow my instructions, you will have amazing results. I promise.

I want you to think, *If not now, when?* When is tomorrow going to happen? Don't you deserve for it to happen now? You have to say, "I'm ready for the Virgin Diet. I'm all in." You can't be a little in on my program. You're either all in or you're not doing this.

So, come on in. I'm here to support you, every step of the way. If you follow my instructions, you will have amazing results. I promise.

# HOW THE VIRGIN DIET WORKED FOR ME

Maggie S.
Age 50

Piscataway,
New Jersey

**Height:**
5'6¾"

**Starting Weight:**
148 pounds

**Waist:** 33.5"
**Hips:** 39"

**Current Weight:**
125 pounds

**Waist:** 27.5"
**Hips:** 36"

**Lost:** 23 pounds

Thanks to the Virgin Diet, I have had tremendous physical changes in my energy and strength. I have been moving a lot more and feel great from feeling strong again. I feel very happy to know that I have been and will continue to feel and look better. This has been a great inspiration to my friends and family. One friend even quit smoking! My sister and I have all kinds of new things to talk about regarding exercise, food and nutrition. I feel a tremendous amount of freedom because I am stronger, and I also feel disciplined, but it is because I want to be, not that I have to be. I understand exactly what I need to do.

I turned 50 last year, and the perimenopause thing really seemed to kick in. Then I was bitten by a brown recluse spider, and it really affected me badly. The poison went to my lungs, kidneys, stomach, all over—plus I had to take antibiotics, which wreaked havoc on my system. I have felt extremely weak since then, and my stomach had been more of a wreck than it usually is. The bite was behind my knee, so I was benched for a few months. As a result,

I gained a bunch of weight and couldn't shake it. I didn't know what to do or where to start.

Enter the Virgin Diet to the rescue! After dropping the 7 foods that JJ recommends we drop, I began to feel better immediately. This whole program has given me my life back. I am actually feeling strong again. JJ's online forum and having a coach have been very supportive in so many ways. I am just beginning to realize the subtleties of that support and how important it is.

The greatest takeaway from this program for me is its comprehensiveness. All aspects are tackled, and I am feeling overall very balanced because of that. I thought the Virgin Diet Shakes were amazing. I really hit the program as hard as I could and have had the blessing of witnessing myself change and transform. This has been a really important experience. I hope I can help others know that transformation is possible and doable and fun!

What advice would I give to others? *Go for it!* Get rid of the 7 foods that JJ talks about immediately, ASAP!!! Make up your mind and follow the guidelines. Get a pedometer and move more. Really get into the bursting and resistance training knowing that they are your best friends! Learn how to really sleep and allow yourself to sleep. Feel excited about starting new healthy habits and breaking old unhealthy habits. The rewards will come!

7 FOODS TO AVOID

# GLUTEN GONE

## 3

My client George had no problem passing on candy, diet soda or ice cream. He didn't have a sweet tooth. Nor did he mind going without butter, cream, rich sauces, fried foods or other types of high-fat choices. When I first told George about the Virgin Diet, he was fine with the idea of giving up sugar and artificial sweeteners, and he didn't think he'd mind letting go of corn, soy, eggs, dairy and peanuts.

Then we got to gluten, and all hell broke loose. Or at least that's what it felt like on my end of the phone as I listened to George vent his frustration.

"No cereal? No granola? No pasta? No couscous? No bread? How do you expect me to do that?"

Gluten is an ingredient found in most grains, especially wheat, barley and rye. It disrupts your digestion by damaging the microvilli of the small intestine, where we absorb our nutrients. Gluten also makes your intestines more permeable, which can lead to leaky gut, food intolerance, immune problems, inflammation and an inability to absorb nutrients and make vitamin B12. What this adds up to is several different ways that gluten causes you to gain weight, which you're then unable to lose.

For some people, gluten is outright dangerous because they have celiac disease, a form of extreme gluten intolerance. If you suffer from celiac disease, the starchy side of life can create serious health risks, including arthritis, osteoporosis and autoimmune conditions. It can even ultimately cause death. Although celiac disease is often hard to diagnose, George's doctor had run tests and already determined that he didn't have it.

Ironically, the one problem that celiac disease does *not* cause is weight gain. Because they have so much difficulty absorbing nutrients, most celiacs are thin or underweight.

Luckily, George did not suffer from this problem. In fact, he was struggling with 20 extra pounds that he wanted to lose.

"If I don't have celiac disease, doesn't that mean it's okay for me to eat gluten?" George asked. "I'm sure I could eat it in moderation, anyway."

"When it comes to gluten—and to the other high-FI foods—moderation doesn't work," I answered. Celiac disease is only the most extreme form of gluten intolerance, just as IgE food allergies are an extreme form of "immune system gone wild." But the less extreme forms can also create significant problems for us. Just because George doesn't have celiac disease didn't mean he couldn't be having other problems with gluten. And if he was, then every time he ate bread, pasta, cereal or baked goods, he was sabotaging his weight-loss efforts—not necessarily because of the calories but because of the way high-FI gluten inflamed his system and disrupted his digestion.

> We've made gluten-containing grains more "gluten-y."

Although celiac disease is relatively rare, gluten problems are much more common, and most people are walking around completely unaware that they are suffering from them. Some 30 to 40 percent of the population, including myself, have some type of gluten issue that also creates symptoms, from joint pain, to brain fog, to gastrointestinal distress. Typically in America, we've made gluten-containing grains more "gluten-y" because it makes them fluffier and softer. If you go to Italy and eat the pasta or pizza, it's entirely different because they haven't overly glutenized their grains.

So, if you've been wondering why bread-loving Italians don't seem to have the same weight problems that we do, that is definitely one of the factors.

"I can't imagine giving up grains," George said finally. He was willing to give up cake. He was willing to give up cereal. But he couldn't stand the thought of giving up bread.

"I understand," I told him. "If I knew I was having my last meal tonight, I'd ask for a loaf of crusty sourdough bread—and I would savor every crumb!

"The problem is, tonight isn't my last meal. I'm going to live a long, long time—or at least I hope I am. If I eat gluten, my digestive system will be all messed up, I'll look old and haggard, I'll develop some medical problems and I'll gain weight. I don't want to live like that—sick and old and fat. Do you?"

There was a silence at the other end of the phone as George thought over what I had said. "Okay," he said finally, "let's give it a try."

## WHAT IS GLUTEN?

**We've been eating gluten all of our lives, often in hidden places.**

Gluten is a form of protein found in wheat, rye, barley and many processed foods. Most of us tend to think, *Oh, proteins—healthy!* But some proteins cause our bodies a world of hurt, and the proteins found in gluten are among the worst culprits.

Yet, we love gluten in this country, which is why you can find it just about everywhere. Gluten in wheat flour makes things light and spongy or chewy and crunchy, and gluten everywhere else acts as a stabilizer and thickening agent, which is why manufacturers add it to such unlikely foods as ice cream, ketchup and mustard. (See the Where Gluten Hides section on page 70.) My guess is that if companies didn't add gluten to so many things, most of us might not have a problem with it because gluten in small amounts is probably okay if you don't have celiac disease. But we've been eating gluten all of our lives, often in hidden places (lunch meats? salad dressings? pickles? *Really?*), so now we have to pass on the pasta and say bye-bye to the bread. I'm sorry, but we do.

Maybe you won't mind letting go of gluten once you learn about all the problems that gluten-bearing foods can cause. Let's take a closer look.

 ## CELIAC DISEASE

If you've heard about problems with gluten, this disease is probably what you heard about. It's relatively rare: only about 1 in 133 people have it, and sadly only a small percentage of them are ever diagnosed.

If you have celiac disease, you cannot eat any gluten. Ever. Period. You've got a genetic condition that won't bother you if you don't consume gluten, but that can set off a major overreaction in your immune system if you *do* eat gluten.

Just the genes and the gluten aren't enough to cause celiac disease, though. You also need a trigger to turn on the problem genes. Common triggers include any type of major trauma to your body, such as surgery, pregnancy or a viral infection, along with something we're all familiar with: stress. So you might have the potential for celiac for years without ever realizing it, and you *may* have been consuming gluten without causing too many problems.

Once celiac disease is triggered, though, that's it. You've got it for life. From that point on, whenever you consume anything that contains gluten, your immune cells immediately try to attack the gluten molecule—and attack your body's cells at the same time. Even if you don't notice any symptoms, your small intestine is taking a hit every time you eat a piece of sourdough rye or grab a granola bar on the go. As a result, you aren't absorbing nutrients properly, and you're facing serious health risks for the future.

Because celiac disease is often misdiagnosed, you could end up eating gluten for years without realizing the harm it is causing to your body. In addition, celiac disease can trigger and exacerbate many of the other 140 autoimmune diseases that we know about. In fact, other autoimmune disorders occur 10 times more often in those with celiac disease than in the general population.

There is no cure for celiac disease, but there is a solution: yank the gluten from your diet. The disease doesn't affect you as long as you're not eating anything that contains gluten.

## GLUTEN SENSITIVITY

**In the United States, 30 to 40 percent of the population has *some* form of sensitivity to gluten.**

Now, here's where things get fuzzy, but hang in there. In the United States, 30 to 40 percent of the population, including me, has *some* form of sensitivity to gluten that is not celiac disease but that is nevertheless a real problem with serious symptoms, including painful digestive problems, headaches, joint pain, infertility, osteoporosis, anxiety or depression. Gluten sensitivity also can damage your intestinal lining and produce leaky gut. And it can vastly increase your chance of gaining weight and making it nearly impossible to lose as long as you keep eating gluten.

If you react badly to gluten but don't test positive for celiac disease, there are two possibilities:

1. **You might actually have celiac disease,** but your testing was done improperly or was insufficient to yield conclusive results. In my personal opinion—shared by a lot of other health experts—celiac disease is way underdiagnosed and is often simply misdiagnosed.

2. **You might not have the genes that cause celiac disease,** but still be highly sensitive to gluten.[8] In his book *Healthier Without Wheat: A New Understanding of Wheat Allergies, Celiac Disease, and Non-Celiac Gluten Intolerance,* Dr. Stephen Wangen, a naturopathic doctor and specialist in food allergies and digestive disorders, has shown that nearly one-third of people who did not have the genetic marker for celiac nonetheless had antigluten antibodies in their stool. These antibodies create the same kinds of problems as the celiac response: a highly reactive immune system that goes after gluten and does a lot of collateral damage to the small intestine at the same time. Interestingly, these antibodies decrease when gluten is removed from the diet.

Unfortunately, much of the traditional medical community still doesn't recognize gluten sensitivity. In most doctors' minds, if it's not outright celiac, it doesn't exist.

In fact, you might not test positive, either for celiac or for any gluten sensitivity. Yet, you yank the gluten and feel a lot better. So, in my opinion, *that's* the best test. If you are eating gluten and feeling bad, what is going on? Something that gluten is doing is causing some kind of inflammatory response in your body. This could be creating other problems as well.

What's the moral of the story? Avoid gluten, at least for the 21 days of Cycle 1. In Cycle 2, we'll find out whether you can tolerate it.

 ## GLUTEN AND LEAKY GUT

What if you have none of these special conditions: celiac disease, a grain allergy, gluten sensitivity or gluten intolerance. *Now* are you off the hook? Nope.

Even among people who have no special sensitivity, gluten triggers the release of a protein called zonulin. I realize that zonulin sounds like the name of a creature from outer space, but it's actually a protein produced in the small intestine. Like any sci-fi villain, zonulin is insidious and potentially quite dangerous, dismantling the proteins that create the tight junctions that we talked about in Chapter 1. Tight junctions are what keep your intestinal lining neatly sealed up so all the partially digested food stays inside. When zonulin messes with those junctions, some of that food leaks out, and your immune system thinks it's being invaded again. Suddenly, you're developing food sensitivities to foods you used to tolerate, and the overall immune response is increasing your level of inflammation. Inflammation causes symptoms plus weight gain.

If the details are too hard to remember, just keep this simple formula in mind:

gluten → leaky gut → food sensitivities →
inflammation + weight gain

That's really all you need to know—and it should inspire you to stay off the gluten.

## GLUTEN PROBLEMS: TEST OR CHALLENGE?

There are some tests you can have for celiac disease and gluten sensitivity. I've listed them in the Resources section on my website so you can ask your doctor about them if you want, but you don't have to go through all of those tests. The simplest way you can check for gluten sensitivity and celiac disease is to not eat it. Pull it out 100 percent, just as we are doing in Cycle 1 of the Virgin Diet. Then, as we are doing in Cycle 2, challenge it back. Then, see how you feel.

I see people all the time who look fine on every single test there is, but they still feel bad. We pull out gluten, and they feel a lot better. Maybe they feel better because they're eating fewer grains (for more on grain problems, see the Lectins and Phytates: The Bad News Twins section later in this chapter). If you don't want to get tested, don't worry. I'll walk you through Cycle 1 and Cycle 2, and that is probably all you need.

## GLUTEN AND AUTOIMMUNE CONDITIONS

Okay, so celiac disease is an autoimmune condition and leaky gut (which can be triggered or worsened by gluten) causes a whole host of problematic immune responses. Autoimmune conditions include asthma, allergies, Hashimoto's thyroiditis (which might also be playing havoc with your weight), rheumatoid arthritis and lupus.

> If you have an autoimmune condition of any kind, the first thing you should do is yank the gluten.

To me, there is one simple conclusion: if you have an autoimmune condition of any kind, the first thing you should do is yank the gluten. It needs to go. I am always amazed at how much we can do to address autoimmunity through nutrition and how little awareness the medical community has of that fact. Too often, practitioners will greet problematic test results with the suggestion to watch closely and see what happens rather than making proactive suggestions about dropping foods that may raise the risk of autoimmunity.

My client Kim had been diagnosed with three separate autoimmune conditions. Her doctor deemed that she was "autoimmune-y" and could offer nothing better than "keep an eye on them." I almost had a heart attack when I heard about it. I knew that anyone who struggles with one autoimmune disease is far more likely to develop another and that Kim's three autoimmune conditions were a strong predictor of her likelihood to develop another—perhaps even several more. As I do with all my autoimmune clients, I immediately got Kim to drop the gluten, dairy and soy from her diet, and I worked with her to make sure she had optimal vitamin D levels. All three of her conditions are virtually asymptomatic now, and she has not gone on to develop any others.

If you have been or are concerned about autoimmunity, get rid of the gluten, dairy and soy, just as I am having you do on this program. You may not be able to cure your condition, but you can definitely keep it from getting worse!

## OPTIMIZE YOUR VITAMIN D

One of the most common triggers for autoimmune diseases is a vitamin D deficiency, so make sure your levels are somewhere in the 60 to 80 ng/ml range. (Your doctor can test your 25-hydroxy vitamin D level.)

### AUTOIMMUNITY AND GLUTEN SENSITIVITY

I've known for a while that gluten sensitivity and autoimmunity were related, but I was blown away by this powerful quote from Peter Osborne, DC, a board-certified doctor in clinical nutrition and a leading expert in gluten intolerance and celiac disease:

> There are actually 140 autoimmune diseases that we've identified, and the only scientifically agreed upon cause for autoimmune is gluten sensitivity. Now there are other triggers for autoimmune disease. An infection can trigger an autoimmune disease. A vitamin deficiency can trigger an autoimmune disease, particularly vitamin D. But gluten tends to be kind of that central core hub that's always present.[9]

Be careful when supplementing, though. When vitamin D is manufactured, gluten and dairy are often used to create the finished product, but ingredients used to make an initial raw ingredient do not need to be noted on the bottle. So, if your supplements make you feel worse, you need to check them out. If you're working with a practitioner who's aware of this issue, find out whether your brands are safe. Otherwise, just buy one of the trusted brands I recommend in the Resources section on my website.

 ## LECTINS AND PHYTATES: THE BAD NEWS TWINS

Gluten-containing grains have both lectins and phytates, which are just bad news. Lectins can bind to insulin receptors, which then creates insulin resistance, which means that your blood sugar rises making it harder to burn off fat. Lectins can also bind to your intestinal lining, which contributes to altered gut flora, causing you to store more calories from the food you eat and, worse yet, store it as fat. Lectins can also be associated with leptin resistance. Because leptin is the hormone that helps regulate feelings of hunger and fullness, leptin resistance makes you hungrier even when you've had all the food you need. It also puts you at risk for metabolic syndrome, the triple threat of obesity, diabetes and high blood pressure. Fun stuff, huh? Take it from me, you don't need the aggravation.

Phytates are equally bad. Found in gluten and other whole grains, we call them the antinutrient because they make minerals bio-unavailable. So much for all those healthy vitamins and minerals we're supposedly getting from whole grains! The whole-grain goodness notion is a fallacy (see page 163 for more on the role of whole grains in the Virgin Diet). If

**The whole-grain goodness notion is a fallacy.**

you really want a small amount of grain in your diet, stick to rice, gluten-free oatmeal, millet, buckwheat and amaranth. You can also choose sweet potatoes, quinoa, lentils and legumes, so don't feel that you need to eat grains to be healthy.

## SOME COOL SUBSTITUTIONS

- **Instead of regular pasta,** try rice pasta, quinoa pasta or spaghetti squash.

- **Instead of tortillas,** try brown rice wraps or large leaves of Romaine lettuce.

- **Instead of wheat or rye flour,** try almond or coconut flour.

- **Instead of soy sauce,** try coconut aminos.

- **Instead of couscous,** try quinoa.

- **Instead of floury pizza crusts,** try a slice of eggplant or a portobello mushroom.

# WHERE GLUTEN HIDES

Gluten is *everywhere,* so read your labels carefully. American strains of wheat have a much higher gluten content than those traditionally found in Europe. This super gluten was recently introduced into our agricultural food supply and has now "infected" nearly all wheat strains in America. Now we have light, fluffy white bread and giant bagels. And gluten lurks in even more places.

# GLUTEN HIDES IN . . .

| | |
|---|---|
| All brans | Muffins |
| Baked beans | Mustard and dry mustard powder |
| Biscuits and cookies | Pancakes |
| Blue cheeses | Pasta (e.g., macaroni and spaghetti) |
| Bread and bread rolls | Pastry and pie crust |
| Breadcrumbs | Pâtés |
| Brown rice syrup | Pizza |
| Bulgur wheat | Pretzels |
| Cakes | Pringles potato chips |
| Cheap brands of chocolate | Pumpernickel |
| Chutneys and pickles | Rye bread |
| Couscous | Sauces (often thickened with flour) |
| Crispbreads | Sausages (often contain rusk) |
| Crumble toppings | Scones |
| Durum | Seitan (doesn't contain gluten, it *is* gluten!) |
| Farina | Self-basting turkeys |
| Gravy powders and stock cubes | Semolina |

| | |
|---|---|
| Hydrolyzed vegetable protein (HVP) | Shredded suet in packs |
| Imitation crabmeat | Some alcoholic drinks |
| Licorice | Some breakfast cereals |
| Luncheon meats (may contain fillers) | Soups (may be roux-based) |
| Malt vinegar | Soy sauce |
| Malted drinks | Spice blends |
| Many salad dressings | Stuffing |
| Matzo flour/meal | Waffles |
| Meat and fish pastes | White pepper |
| Muesli | Yorkshire pudding |

## WHAT'S LURKING IN YOUR LUNCH MEATS?

Many lunch meats are injected with gluten. I guess that's because it's so good at stabilizing and thickening, but it's probably also why so many of us have developed gluten sensitivity. So make sure your lunch meat is gluten-free, or pick up fresh, gluten-free foods instead, such as fresh chicken or wild salmon. If you need "grab and go" protein, consider some gluten-free, grass-fed beef jerky or an aseptic pack of wild salmon. They are healthier choices for many other reasons, too.

## OATMEAL: OUT OR IN?

Oatmeal itself is gluten-free, so in theory, you should be able to eat anything made with oats (as long as it doesn't contain dairy, eggs or gluten!). However, oatmeal is often made in places where they also process grains that *do* contain gluten, and there is a great deal of cross-contamination. So make sure you're buying only oatmeal that is marked "gluten-free." (You can find a list of brands in the Resources section on my website.)

# WHEN GLUTEN-FREE ISN'T GOOD FOR YOU

Now that more and more people are realizing the dangers of gluten, a whole new line of gluten-free products has come on the market. This can be a problem, though, because a lot of these foods aren't healthy and can lead to weight gain—even if they are gluten-free!

In fact, gluten-free has become the new faux health food. There are gluten-free cookies, breads and muffins. Most of those are loaded with sugar. *Gluten-free* does not necessarily mean healthy— and it *definitely* does not mean good for weight loss.

> **If you're looking at a food that's completely processed, it is not healthy.**

I've had clients who went along with my recommendation to pull all the gluten out of their diets, and all of a sudden they're gorging themselves on gluten-free bread, muffins, cookies and cakes. I say, "Hey, you didn't eat this stuff before! Why are you eating it now?"

I don't care where you found it or what the label says, if you're looking at a food that's completely processed, it is not healthy. A rice cake, bread, cookie, muffin or cracker might be gluten-free, but it's processed, so leave it, all right?

Do you want some *real* gluten-free goodness? The very best gluten-free foods come in their own natural packaging. Some of my favorite examples are apples, broccoli, sweet potatoes and avocados.

 ## GLUTEN-FREE GOODNESS

When you remove the gluten from the diet of someone who is gluten-sensitive, you can get near-miraculous results. My client Petra had suffered for a year with chronic tendinitis. She had seen numerous physical therapists, plus MDs, acupuncturists and pain specialists. None of them could make much of a difference in her condition, and in fact, the pain was getting worse.

Then, she gave up gluten for 1 week, and suddenly all of her pain was gone. If I hadn't seen it myself—and if I hadn't experienced a miniversion of her experience with my own gluten-induced swollen fingers—I'm not sure I would have believed it.

Petra is not my only client to experience such dramatic responses to a gluten-free diet, not to mention the countless men and women who simply feel better when they don't consume it. George, my client who couldn't bear to give up bread, was actually delighted to discover how much better he felt on a gluten-free regime.

"I just feel clearer and more focused," he told me when we last met. "And I've definitely got more energy. Plus, I have to admit, cutting out gluten made it a lot easier to lose weight!"

"It's hard to get in trouble when you pull gluten out," I agreed. "No pizza, no baked goods, no pasta, no bread—a lot of weight-loss obstacles are just out the window."

George laughed. "I remember how I thought I could never live without gluten," he told me. "And now, to be honest, I can't even imagine eating it again. Who could have thought that gluten-free would feel so good?"

Bill Nardiello
Age 63

Dallas,
Texas

**Height:**
5'9"

**Starting Weight:**
175 pounds

**Waist:** 35"
**Hips:** 38"

**Current Weight:**
160 pounds

**Waist:** 33.5"
**Hips:** 37"

**Lost:** 15 pounds

# HOW THE VIRGIN DIET WORKED FOR ME

For my entire life, I had intestinal issues that doctors were not able to diagnose. For decades, doctors dealt with my symptoms with no clue as to the cause.

Then I met JJ, who had me pull gluten and eggs out of my diet. I was skeptical at the beginning, but then my symptoms disappeared almost immediately. I was so excited to finally have an answer to my health problems! I was grateful beyond words that JJ understood what was wrong with me and could help me find a solution that actually worked.

Any time I add in gluten or eggs, I immediately get the same symptoms that I had before. But when I leave them out of my diet, my energy is better, I sleep better and my overall health is excellent.

Thanks to JJ, my life changed dramatically. I had accepted my physical lot in life as something I just had to live with, and I never really expected to find a solution.

I still can't believe what a difference it made to pull out these so-called "healthy" foods that were almost killing me. Pulling out these problem foods changed my life.

# NO JOY IN SOY

## 4

I get lots of letters and e-mails from men and women who discover my website, see me on television or attend one of my lectures. But the following, hands down, has got to be one of the most moving e-mails I have ever received:

Dear JJ:

When I went to your lecture, I was 100 pounds overweight. I swear I never ate sugar. I was practically a vegan. I lived on soy and other foods I truly thought were healthy. But I could never lose weight—never. It was making me crazy because I didn't understand what I was doing wrong.

Then I went to your lecture, and I'll be honest, I took one look at you and hated you on sight. I thought, *She is thin and beautiful. What does she have to tell me about losing weight? She doesn't understand.*

But then you started talking about food intolerance, and you mentioned soy, and I realized, oh, my God, you do understand. In fact, you were describing me exactly. I was eating "healthy" foods every day—and they were making me sick and keeping me fat. I started crying. The woman next to me—a total stranger—had to hold my hand all the way through your lecture.

I have cut out the soy. I have dropped the other 6 high-FI foods. And I have started losing weight! I have discovered I had a thyroid condition that the soy was aggravating, and that was both keeping me fat and piling on the symptoms. That's all much better. I can't believe how much energy I have and how good I feel!

I haven't just changed my body, I've changed my life. I feel good and confident and energized, and it inspired me to quit my job working for a headhunting firm and work for myself, as a business coach. I have more clients than I can handle—and enough energy to handle them! I feel great, I think I look great, and I'm really happy. *Thank you* for giving me the key to my health.

With all my thanks—Bryn

I was so happy to help Bryn—and I was so glad to get the word out about soy. Although there is so much propaganda out there about how healthy soy is, the truth is much more disturbing. Although you might be able to tolerate small amounts of organic fermented soy, you certainly shouldn't be eating soy in large amounts—and, like Bryn, you might not be able to tolerate any soy at all. Let's take a closer look.

 # DON'T BELIEVE THE HYPE

Unless you've been living in a cave the past 15 years, you've heard the hype: soy is the new miracle food that helps your heart and makes you healthy. Don't believe it. The health benefits of soy have been greatly exaggerated, mostly by the soy industry itself.

NO JOY IN SOY

Here are just some of the key problems with soy:

- **It disrupts your hormones.** Soy is what's known as a *phyto-estrogen*—a plant source of the hormone estrogen. The jury is still out on whether soy is a positive or a negative for women, but it definitely isn't good for children or men.

> The health benefits of soy have been greatly exaggerated, mostly by the soy industry itself.

- **It's bad for your thyroid.** Chronic soy consumption may impair thyroid function, which, as Bryn found out, makes it nearly impossible to lose weight.

- **It's new to the food supply.** Generally, the stuff we've been eating for our entire history on the planet is healthier than the food items we've added to our diets more recently.

- **It's genetically modified.** The new trend of genetically modifying vast amounts of our food supply is one of the scariest developments in recent years, and the soy crop is one of the most genetically modified there is—more than 90 percent, by most estimates.

- **It's overly processed.** Usually, the more processed a food has been, the more it's been stripped of vital nutrients. That equals empty calories—and why do that to your body?

Now, if you don't react to soy and don't have thyroid or estrogen issues, you can incorporate a small amount of fermented soy into your diet, but only organic, please, and not daily—just a couple times a week. But we won't know whether it's okay to put soy back in until we take it out. So, for Cycle 1, I want you to be 100 percent soy-free.

I'd also like you to understand my concerns—and my colleagues' concerns—about this problematic food. By the time you've finished this chapter, I want you to be 100 percent clear about why I find no joy in soy.

## SOY: THE SHAM HEALTH FOOD

Soy has been marketed as the miracle food of all time, maybe because it can be produced cheaply and some big companies have invested in its production and modification. If you go to Natural Products Expo West and other big health-food conventions, they can seem like one big homage to soy.

Yet, eating soy on a daily basis may create problems, whether in traditional forms like tofu and edamame or in more modern incarnations, such as soy milk, soy ice cream and soy cheese.

**Soy can be an *anti*nutrient.**

One study showed that high midlife tofu consumption—high being only 2 servings per week—increased the risk of late-life cognitive impairment and dementia in both men and women.[10] Another study, published by Hogervorst and his colleagues, showed that tofu intake was associated with poor memory and dementia in a group of 700 older adults.[11]

Soy is rich in phytates, or phytic acid, which blocks the absorption of minerals, especially calcium, magnesium, copper, iron and zinc. In other words, soy can be an *anti*nutrient. To neutralize the phytates in soy, you'd have to ferment the heck out of it, as they do in Asia. That is not how most of our soy is prepared here.

Soy is also full of trypsin inhibitors. Trypsin is an enzyme produced in the pancreas that we need to digest protein. Trypsin inhibitors can interfere with protein digestion and cause pancreatic disorders. Not surprisingly, in countries where there is more soy consumption, we find more pancreatic, stomach and thyroid cancers.

Soy promoters will tell you that soy is good for osteoporosis. But as we just saw, the phytates in soy can impair calcium and magnesium absorption. So how is that good for your bones? Soy also increases the body's need for vitamin D. Often, vitamin D2, also known as ergocalciferol, will be added to soy milk. However, the preferred form of vitamin D is D3, or cholecalciferol. This is the form of vitamin D that humans synthesize from sunlight. It is more potent and stable than D2, raises blood levels of vitamin D longer and binds to vitamin D receptors better—but it's not usually found in soy milk, even as soy increases your body's need for it. So, in all those senses, soy can be bad for bone health.

> The phytates in soy can impair calcium and magnesium absorption.

What about soy as a source of protein? Again, the news is not good. Although soy is a complete protein, it has very low amounts of two essential amino acids, lysine and methionine, so it is not a quality protein source.

You might have heard reports that modern soy foods offer protection against some types of cancer. However, according to a 2002 report by the United Kingdom Food Standards Agency's Committee on Toxicity, there's not much evidence for that. Soy foods might even result in an increased risk of certain cancers.

Now, there is *some* evidence that soy lowers cholesterol. However, I am still not convinced that lowering cholesterol reduces your risk for heart disease. In any case, there are far better ways to lower cholesterol, including lowering your overall glycemic load, getting rid of damaged fats and increasing your intake of fiber.

If you've been keeping score, you can see that there are lots of reasons to avoid soy and really no reason at all to consume it. Unfortunately, there are a lot more soy negatives still to come.

## YOU ARE WHAT YOU EAT, ATE

Sometimes you think you've done all there is to do, and then one of those sneaky high-FI foods makes it into your diet anyway. For example, I once had a very soy-sensitive client who had cut out all the soy—we thought—and she was still getting sick. We wondered where the heck it was coming from.

It turned out that she had been buying chicken—from a well-known health-food store, mind you!—and those chickens had been fed soy. People say, "You are what you eat," but I say, "You are what you eat, ate." It is challenging because most chickens, even the naturally raised ones, have their diet supplemented with corn and/or soy. Fortunately, unless you are highly sensitive to soy or corn, this won't create a problem for you, but ideally you will want to seek out the cleanest sources of poultry you can find. Make friends with your local farmers or check out U.S. Wellness Meats (see the Resources section on my website).

## THE TRUTH ABOUT SOY IN ASIA

Now, at this point you might be thinking, *But they eat a lot of soy in Asia, and isn't it good for people's health there?*

For millennia, the Asians used soy as a fertilizer crop. They rotated it in between the plantings of their regular crops because it replenished the soil with nitrogen, much like fertilizer does. Then, someone discovered that if you fermented soybeans, you could overcome a lot of their antinutrient properties. So Asians began consuming fermented soy, but not a lot of it. Having lived in Japan, I can tell you that I never saw anyone eat soy ice cream, soy cheese, soy hot dogs, soy burgers, soy pops or soy milk. True, soy is part of the traditional Asian diet, but they do not eat a big pile of it. You have a little miso soup, some tofu in a stir-fry or some soy sauce with your sushi. You don't drink a big soy shake in the morning, have a soy yogurt at lunch and have soy cheese or tofu stir-fry at dinner.

Basically, in Asia, soy is a condiment. It is *not* a replacement for animal proteins.

Plus, the soy in Asia is organic—no GMOs and no chemicals in the fertilizer. And Asian soy is very fermented, which helps reduce phytates and lectins. That is a very different way to use soy. Yes, if you ate soy the way they do in Asia—in small, organic, fermented amounts—it would probably be okay. But living in the United States, that is nearly impossible to do, and just about all of our soy crop has been genetically modified. I'll get to that in a minute. First, I want to get to some other health concerns.

## SOY DISRUPTS YOUR HORMONES

Let's start with sex hormones. For both men and women, this is kind of a scary topic. Researchers are still trying to figure out whether soy stimulates cancer cells—especially breast cancer cells—and the growth of estrogen-dependent tumors. We don't yet know, but we do know that soy is a phytoestrogen—a plant source of estrogen. That means that it can disrupt hormone balances for both genders.

For women, depending on how much you eat, soy can affect ovulation. Although phytoestrogens are being touted as good for postmenopausal women, there is not yet any clear proof to show that this is the case.

As for men, how can all that estrogen be good for them? I don't think it is. Soy can lower testosterone in men. In fact, there's an old wives' tale in Japan that when women are worried about their husbands' fidelity, they feed their men soy—to keep them from fooling around. I don't know about that, but we do see more infertility with excessive soy consumption. Soy has also been linked to infertility in animals.

Soy can also affect children's development, thanks to its hormonal effects. Boys' genitals may not develop fully, and little girls may develop faster and start their menses earlier than normal. You don't want to feed soy to infants either. It can impact brain and nervous system development.

## SOY IS BAD FOR YOUR THYROID

Bryn found out this sad truth the hard way: soy can depress thyroid function. I've seen this often among my clients. When they eat soy every day, they tend to have elevated levels of TSH (thyroid-stimulating hormone), which is an indicator of hypothyroidism. Then I see their thyroid numbers come back to normal quickly when soy is taken out of their diets.

Depending on how much you've tweaked your thyroid already, you might need some extra support for getting it back in shape, so I suggest you talk to your doctor. Make sure your doctor runs the full panel of thyroid tests. Many general practitioners and endocrinologists only run tests for TSH and T4, the inactive thyroid. You also need to be tested for free T3 (the active thyroid hormone, which is converted from T4) and thyroid antibodies so you get a full picture of what's going on.

You want to test the antibodies because, sad to say, soy can trigger an autoimmune condition in which your body makes antibodies that attack your thyroid hormone. As a result, even if your thyroid gland is making enough of this vital biochemical, your body doesn't get what it needs because the antibodies are destroying it. A high level of thyroid antibodies often indicates some kind of autoimmune condition.

I have heard many clients say, "My thyroid antibodies were high. We're going to watch them." That's not what you want to do. If you see a high level of antibodies, you need to pull out all the potentially reactive foods immediately. When you pull out gluten, dairy and soy, the antibodies often come down quickly. Luckily, with the Virgin Diet, that is what you're doing anyway.

Soy's impact is all the more problematic because it's not the only factor that can affect thyroid function or disrupt the conversion of inactive T4 to active T3. Other disrupters include heavy metal toxicity, nutritional deficiencies and poor iodine status. Aging can be a factor, as can genetics. And of course, our old friend stress has a big role to play, too.

Finally, soy has been linked to thyroid cancer and to autoimmune thyroid disease in infants drinking soy formula. You can see why I'm concerned about you eating soy.

## HYPOTHYROID: COMMON SYMPTOMS

| | |
|---|---|
| Congested skin or acne | Low libido |
| Constipation | Memory problems |
| Depression | Menstrual irregularities |
| Dry, brittle nails | Puffiness |
| Elevated cholesterol | Rough, itchy, thinning or dry skin |
| Enlarged neck | Slowed thinking |
| Exhaustion | Sluggishness |
| Feeling cold | Thinning outer third of the eyebrows |
| Hair loss, thinning or dry hair | Weight gain |
| Inability to sweat | Yellowish tinge on skin |
| Infertility | |

If you show any of these signs, consult an integrative physician. See the Resources section on my website for some suggestions on how to find one.

## SOY IS NEW TO THE FOOD SUPPLY

Now, for another clue as to why soy isn't ideal food for us, let's look at what humans have been eating since we showed up on the planet. For hundreds of thousands of years, we were hunters and gatherers. We ate raw nuts and seeds, wild animals that were not domesticated or fed grain, wild fish and insects. (Don't worry, there are no insects on the Virgin Diet!) We also ate fruits and vegetables, depending on the season. If we could find an egg, we ate it, too—but that didn't happen on a consistent basis.

Then, 5,000 to 10,000 years ago, we introduced grains into our diet. We also started keeping domesticated animals, which meant that some cultures were eating dairy and eggs on a regular basis. A lot of nutritional experts argue that this is why many of us have trouble digesting grains, dairy and eggs—we just haven't had time for our bodies to adapt to that way of eating.

In any case, soy came into our food supply only 2,000–3,000 years ago. Although this might seem like a long time, when you're looking at how long we've been on the planet, it's really just a moment. And even that figure is deceptive because we've only been consuming soy as part of our typical diet for the past 20 to 30 years, when we started to go low-carb and subbed in soy for grains.

Frankly, I think the main reason that soy has become a super health food is because it is so cheap to produce. Why? It's cheap partly because of the way it's been genetically modified.

# SOY HAS BEEN GENETICALLY MODIFIED

Basically, soy is cheap because the big companies have figured out how to genetically modify it so it can be sprayed with a potent herbicide that kills everything around it without destroying the soy crop.

Farmers can now plant a ton of soy and spray the heck out of it. So, where is that poison going? Into the soybeans—and then into the person who consumes the soy. Or, if the soy is fed to cattle or farm-raised fish, which is becoming more and more common, then the poison goes into those animals and *then* into you. Remember, you are what you eat, ate.

GMOs are also seriously damaging our gut health because when we eat these genetically modified crops, the altered genes are absorbed by the bacteria in our guts, which changes our gut flora. As a result, we are setting up our intestinal flora to be resistant to antibiotics.

Furthermore, because GMO crops are built to withstand pesticides, they are more heavily sprayed than non-GMO crops. So, GMO crops are responsible for putting more poison into our air, earth and water—and our bodies.

I don't think it's an accident that just when genetically modified foods flooded the market—between 1994 and 2001—food-related illnesses doubled. Genetically modified foods tend to be more allergenic, antinutritional, carcinogenic and toxic, with special dangers for your gastrointestinal tract, your endocrine system and your immune system. So we're going to see more infertility, immune issues and gastrointestinal changes.

Animals that have been fed genetically modified foods have been known to have bleeding stomachs, damaged organs and immune system problems. The animals themselves often have infertility problems, miscarriages and premature births. Their young suffer from lower birth weights, inability to reproduce and altered DNA functioning. If that's what's happening to them, what's happening to us?

In my view, genetically altered foods are anything but innocuous. When you start to create new genes, you have no idea what the result will be.

The American Academy of Environmental Medicine recommends that we avoid genetically modified food. They think it's very dangerous, and so do I. And so do many parts of Western Europe, where genetically modified foods have been outlawed. In the Resources section on my website, I've included leading GMO expert Jeffrey Smith's website, and you can also go to www.thevirgindiet.com/GMO to listen to an interview I did with him. For the sake of your weight, your health and your children's health, stay away from GMOs.

## GMOs AND *SEEDS OF DECEPTION*

I first realized how dangerous and unhealthy GMOs are when I listened to a lecture given at the American College of Alternative Medicine by Jeffrey Smith. He is the author of *Seeds of Deception: Exposing Industry and Government Lies About the Safety of the Genetically Engineered Foods You're Eating,* a pioneering book that was one of the first to document the problems with genetically modified foods. He has been researching GMOs for years, and so far he has documented 65 serious health risks from them. For example, he has found that offspring of rats that were fed genetically modified soy suffered a fivefold increase in mortality along with lower birth weights and the inability to reproduce. Male mice fed genetically modified soy had abnormal sperm counts. Smith also found that many farmers have seen sterility or infertility problems in animals fed genetically modified corn or soy.

## SOY HAS BEEN OVERLY PROCESSED AND REFINED

Refined soy—soy hot dogs, soy ice cream, soy yogurt, soy milk—is even more problematic. Most of these soy "foods" are incredibly refined products with sugar added. So the first thing you have to ask yourself is, *Does eating refined foods versus whole foods make sense?*

Now let's look at *how* soy is processed: it's spun in aluminum casks. That means refined soy can also contain aluminum, which is bad for your health in countless ways, plus MSG is added to improve the taste, which increases soy's reactivity for a lot of people. You should also know that if an item is put in during processing, it might not necessarily be listed in the finished product's ingredients. That means you don't really know *what* you're getting.

> Soy is not the health food it is touted to be.

So, you get it, right? Soy is not the health food it is touted to be—not when you consume it as edamame, and much less so when you eat it as ice cream. During Cycle 1, let's take it out 100 percent. We'll see about putting it back—in small quantities—during Cycle 2.

## WHERE SOY HIDES

| | | |
|---|---|---|
| Asian foods | Soy protein powders | Teriyaki sauce |
| Energy bars and shakes | Soy sauce | Textured vegetable protein |
| Miso | Tempeh | Tofu |
| Prepared foods | | Veggie burgers |

## LOVE THE LECITHIN

The one form of soy that is just fine to eat is soy lecithin, a common ingredient in many gluten-free and vegan breakfast shakes, protein bars and other such foods. This ingredient is all right because it is protein-free—and it is the protein that sparks the allergies.

John Johnson
Age 47

Decatur,
Georgia

**Height:**
5'9"

**Starting Weight:**
211.5 pounds

**Current Weight:**
199 pounds

**Lost:** 12.5 pounds

# HOW THE VIRGIN DIET WORKED FOR ME

The Virgin Diet works! The last time I was below 200 was 4 years ago. I think of losing weight like holding one's breath: you can only do it for so long. I could only starve myself for so long, and then bam! I'd gain it all back. Well, not this time. I was so excited when I saw the 199 on my scale that I couldn't believe it!

You don't need to spend a lot of money to go on the Virgin Diet or deprive yourself. I can stay on it indefinitely—and not eat plastic food from cardboard boxes either.

I was so lucky to find JJ Virgin! I now know how to eat in restaurants. I now cook great meals for my family. My wife lost 4 pounds in 1 week, just eating the healthy meals I made for her. I save a ton of money by not buying dinners out, and I'm not tempted to overeat. The recipes are simple and quick to make.

If you want to get in shape, eat right and feel great, this is the program for you.

# DUMP THE DAIRY

## 5

"JJ, it's just not fair!" my client Michele exclaimed. "No one should have to tolerate both wrinkles and acne!"

Michele and I shared a laugh over her mock-desperate tone, but I knew that for Michele, the problem of acne was not only real but also serious. A professional speaker and author who was a frequent guest on talk shows, Michele was always in the public eye, and her appearance was obviously a significant part of her professional life. As a result, her frequent skin breakouts were driving her to distraction. She had tried covering them up with makeup, but of course, that didn't really hide anything and only made the problem worse.

"There is a solution, Michele," I assured her. "I can give it to you in three words: dump the dairy."

If you love Greek-style yogurt, foamy milk on your cappuccino or goat cheese on your salad, you won't be happy to hear those words. However, if you want healthy, glowing skin, you will be delighted with the results you get with the Virgin Diet. Many of the 7 high-FI foods are bad for your skin, but dairy in particular causes problem after problem. Dairy contains hormones that turn on oil glands, and it's a big reason for our current upswing in adult acne.

We've all heard the propaganda pushing dairy as a super health food, but in fact, cow's milk can be so bad for skin that when I'm working

> **Even people who can tolerate dairy might still be having problems with it.**

with a client battling acne, rosacea or any other skin condition, the first thing I do is tell them to dump the dairy.

Many people are also lactose-intolerant—lacking the enzymes needed to digest dairy—but even people who can tolerate dairy might still be having problems with it. Dairy is one of the most common sources of both food sensitivity and food allergy, sending our immune systems into an uproar with each spoonful of yogurt or sip of milk. If you are sensitive to dairy, you'll likely have acne, rosacea, mucus problems, gas and bloating or sinusitis.

To be sure, these problems might diminish or even disappear after you've had 21 days of freedom from the top 7 high-FI foods. So when we get to Cycle 2, we'll challenge dairy back in and find out whether you can have some occasionally or perhaps even on a regular basis.

Meanwhile, even if you can tolerate dairy, there are several significant problems that it can create for you. Here are some of my biggest concerns:

- It can make you fat.
- It can promote insulin resistance (which contributes to weight gain).
- It can cause or exacerbate acne and other skin problems.
- It can be bad for your bones. (Yes, you heard me. Because of its acidity, dairy might actually *contribute* to osteoporosis.)

Ready to learn more? I know dairy products can be tempting, but once you know the effects they have on your body, you may find them just a little easier to resist.

# DAIRY MAKES YOU FAT

Now, I know what some of you are thinking. You are remembering that study that was blasted all over the media saying that eating dairy could help you lose weight. Although studies have shown this, it's noteworthy that they were all led by the same researcher. However, several studies have tried to replicate those findings, and none of them have succeeded. So, despite all the hype, that study does not look very promising at this point, especially since there is more research out there showing just the opposite: if you drink more milk, you *gain* weight.[12]

> If you drink more milk, you *gain* weight.

Remember when you were growing up and your teacher showed you the food pyramid, the one that told you to drink a lot of milk? Well, a recent study led by Dr. Walter Willet at Harvard's School of Public Health found that children who drink 3 servings of skim or 1 percent milk each day—as opposed to higher fat dairy products—were more prone to becoming overweight than the children who drank fewer such servings each day. The study, conducted by mail-in questionnaires, included 12,829 children ages 9 to 14—a huge and therefore highly significant study.

Although the children's weight gain may have been due to the increase in calories, the weight gain was only associated with skim and 1 percent milk rather than with full-fat dairy products. Possibly this was due to the higher relative lactose content of lower fat milk—remember, lactose is a type of sugar—or perhaps it was due to the hormones and other growth factors in milk, which are higher in concentration when fat content is lower.[13]

## DAIRY MAKES YOU GROW

So let's look more closely at those growth factors, which I bet is something you never even consider when you think about milk, let alone yogurt, cheese or whey. But now I want you to think about it: what is dairy for? Basically, it exists to help baby animals grow bigger, right? As a result, every mother's milk is full of natural anabolic hormones, or growth hormones, such as IGF-1, an insulin-like growth factor.

Hormone-free milk does not exist. Even the most organic, pure and natural milk is basically a delivery vehicle for hormones—vital chemicals intended to spur growth. When we're grown-up, however, that same mother's milk can help us get fat and develop acne.

## DAIRY PROMOTES INSULIN RESISTANCE

Here's another one of dairy's weight-related problems: insulin resistance. As we saw in Chapter 1, this is what occurs when your body is given too much sugar to break down at once.

Now here's where it gets complicated: even though it's low on the glycemic index, dairy affects insulin secretion. (The glycemic index measures how quickly a food converts into blood sugar and how intense the insulin response needs to be as a result. See pages 128–129 for more information on this.) So when people consume dairy products, they can suffer from elevated insulin and insulin resistance.

# DAIRY GIVES YOU ACNE

When you raise insulin and throw in a few growth factors, what do you get? You guessed it: you get acne. I take this one very personally because I struggled a lot with acne when I was growing up. My doctors always told me it was fine to eat dairy products, but now I know that all dairy products, including yogurt, cheese and ice cream, contain hormones that turn on the oil glands, and it could be contributing to our current upswing in adult acne.

One of the largest and longest studies of women's health is the Nurses' Health Study, which looked at some 77,761 nurses over 12 years. Guess what they found? Those who drank more milk as teenagers had higher rates of severe teenage acne than those who drank less. Here's the shocker: skim milk was worse than the full-fat milk. It turns out that when you take the fat out of the milk, you're left with more lactose, which is another word for milk sugar. Any type of sugar is bad for acne, so that may be one of the reasons. The researchers also hypothesized that the presence of hormones and bioactive molecules in the milk might have been the cause.[14]

# DAIRY IS BAD FOR YOUR BONES

Now, I want you to take care of your bone health, but I don't want you to do so by relying on dairy. Why? The Nurses' Health Study also showed that those who had the highest milk consumption had the highest risk of bone fractures. This was a 12-year prospective study among 77,761 women ages 34 through 59 who had never used calcium supplements. Researchers concluded that the study data didn't support the hypothesis that higher consumption of milk or other food sources of calcium protected against hip or forearm fractures.[15] If you look at countries with the highest milk consumption, they also tend to have the highest levels of osteoporosis, so there must be a connection.

## DUMP THE DAIRY, KEEP THE CALCIUM

You do need good sources of calcium for optimal bone health and good health in general. Here are my top 10 bone health foods:

1. Flaxseeds
2. Spinach
3. Sardines
4. Walnuts
5. Brazil nuts
6. Greens (e.g., collard and mustard)
7. Sesame seeds
8. Wild salmon
9. Broccoli
10. Kale

## CRAVING THE DAIRY

Even when you know about all these problems, it can be hard to dump the dairy. In my experience, dairy products are some of the hardest for my clients to give up—and to be honest, they were pretty painful for me to let go of, too. They taste delicious, they show up everywhere, and for many of us, they are part of our earliest memories of comfort food: a warm cup of hot cocoa, a gooey grilled-cheese sandwich, a creamy serving of macaroni and cheese. Even the more adult versions—tangy

Greek-style yogurt, a little blue cheese on a salad, that one inch of foamy milk on a latte—are still seductive.

But you know, sometimes the things we crave are not just the things that make us feel good, they're also the things we're addicted to. As we've seen, when you develop reactivity to a food, your immune system produces this whole special set of antibodies that are custom designed to seek out that food and zap it. That creates a craving—we "want" the food so our antibodies can destroy it. The more reactive you are to dairy—and it is one of the most reactive foods—the more antibodies you've built up and the more intense your craving.

There is another possibly addictive factor here: casein, the protein found in milk and other dairy products. We know that casein can have a morphine-like effect in the brain. In fact, when you consume casein, your body actually produces casomorphins, which have the same physically soothing properties that morphine and other drugs have. So when you feel calmer and happier after eating that macaroni and cheese, that's not just a psychological reaction. It's also a biological reaction. Even whey protein, which is derived from dairy, might have a little bit of casein, which is why you might find yourself craving that cool whey shake.

When that craving hits, remember all those symptoms. And remember that creating all those antibodies and then giving them more of their favorite enemy to zap is not actually good for your body, even though it feels good. Your immune system shouldn't go on high alert every time you pick up a container of yogurt. We want to save it for the real enemies. That temporary casomorphin high is just not worth it.

## DAIRY AND AUTOIMMUNITY

I find it interesting that dairy can also trigger autoimmune diseases. For example, it has been linked to multiple sclerosis.[16] My feeling about dairy and autoimmune conditions is pretty much the same as my feeling about soy: if you have any kind of autoimmune condition, if your antinuclear antibodies (ANAs) are high, or if you have a family history of autoimmune disease (putting you at risk for an autoimmune condition), dump the dairy.

> Dairy can also trigger autoimmune diseases.

## LACTOSE INTOLERANCE

About 75 percent of the worldwide population is lactose-intolerant—that is, most people in the world don't have the enzymes they need to digest lactose found in dairy products. The U.S. rate of lactose intolerance is 25 percent, and anyone from any ethnicity might have it. Symptoms of lactose intolerance are not fun. They include gas, bloating, cramps and diarrhea, as well as itchy skin, eczema, wheezing, congestion, runny nose and watery eyes.

## DISCONTENTED COWS

At this point, honestly, it's hard to tell which dairy problems come from the milk itself and which are the result of the atrocious way we treat our cows. Maybe in some ideal, alternate, organic universe—or even just 50 years ago—we could all be eating our dairy in peace and quiet. But the way today's cows are treated—and then, the way today's milk is treated—creates a whole host of new problems.

First, these days, just about all of our milk is pasteurized by law. Pasteurization is a process that kills bacteria, which includes some bad bacteria that we don't want. But it also destroys the good bacteria that we *do* want, as well as some other vital ingredients in the milk: probiotics, vitamins and enzymes. Basically, to me, pasteurization creates a dead food. (It is very difficult to get raw cow's milk and cheese, depending on the rules in your state. If you can get some, it's definitely worth it. Check the Resources section on my website to find out what might be available in your area.)

Today, manufacturers have to pasteurize milk to counteract the ill effects of keeping cows in close confinement and then feeding them genetically modified corn. The corn causes acidosis, an acid overload in the cows that can produce ulcers and bleeding in the stomach. For this, the cows must be treated with antibiotics, which then go into *our* systems, making it more likely that we won't respond well to antibiotics when we really need them and creating all sorts of antibiotic-resistant bacteria. Meanwhile, though, the bacteria problem also requires that the milk be pasteurized.

Besides antibiotics, cows are often given rBGH, recombinant bovine growth hormone, a genetically modified hormone that basically forces them to give milk far more often than nature ever intended. A cow given rBGH produces 15 times as much milk as a natural cow.

Think about it for a moment. Cows aren't supposed to give milk year-round at high doses. No calf needs that much milk. Only people consuming excessive amounts of dairy products need that much milk. We are essentially forcing cows to produce more milk than they ever would naturally.

The rBGH is bad for the cows and bad for us. First, rBGH amplifies levels of IGF-1, a growth hormone that promotes cancerous tumors in the breast, colon and prostate. As a result of all the extra milking, the cows tend to get infected udders, which requires antibiotic treatment and creates more pus in the milk.

In other words, the cows were producing more milk but lower quality milk. They didn't have a rest period. They didn't have time to rebuild and get the nutrients back that they needed. So we're looking at a liquid with extra hormones, lots of dead pus cells and a whole load of antibiotics. Is that something you want to put inside your body? I didn't think so.

 ## GRASS-FED VERSUS CORN-FED COWS

Now, even though the milk from grass-fed cows is usually pasteurized, you're starting with a whole other product. There's a huge difference between grass-fed pastured cows and cows that are fed genetically modified corn and closely confined. That second group is getting that acid load, plus they're living in conditions that are so unhealthy that they need those massive doses of antibiotics. Cows who feed on grass are much healthier.

Another great thing about grass-fed cows is that both their meat and their milk have a different essential fatty acid blend. In fact, it's an ideal blend, with 5 times more conjugated linoleic acid (CLA). CLA is a great fatty acid that helps you burn off belly fat and may reduce the risk of cancer. Grass-fed raw cow's milk is also high in beta-carotene, vitamin A and vitamin E. With pasture-fed cows, you will see rich, yellow dairy products. This is because of the carotenoids, the same ingredient that gives carrots and squash their brilliant golden color.

That said, most of those good ingredients will be destroyed when you pasteurize the milk. Basically, you're left with fat, sugar and some vitamins and minerals—but not nearly as many as our ancestors got when *they* drank milk.

## WHERE DAIRY HIDES

Butter and many margarines

Chocolate (except some dark chocolate products)

Cottage cheese

Cow's, goat's and sheep's milk, yogurts and cheeses

Cream, sour cream, half-and-half and whipped cream

Cream soups and chowders

Creamy cheese or butter sauces
(often served on vegetables and meats)

Creamy soups and sauces

Ice cream

Macaroni and cheese

Many baked goods (bread, crackers and desserts)

Many baking mixes and pancake mix

Many canned foods (e.g., soups, spaghetti and ravioli)

Many salad dressings (e.g., ranch, blue cheese, creamy and Caesar)

Mashed potatoes (often prepared with butter and/or milk)

Shakes and hot chocolate mixes and drinks

Whey protein powder

### DAIRY MAY BE LISTED ON LABELS AS:

Butter or artificial butter flavor

Buttermilk or buttermilk solids

Casein, caseinate or sodium caseinate

Cheese, cream cheese or cottage cheese

Lactose or lactalbumin

Milk, milk solids or nonfat milk solids

Whey

Yogurt or kefir

## SOME COOL SUBSTITUTIONS

Instead of regular butter, you can enjoy ghee, or clarified butter, ideally from grass-fed cows. Because ghee has no milk solids, you can have it even in Cycle 1.

You should also discover the wonders of coconut milk. If we would all just trade cows for coconuts, I think we'd be a lot better off! I am a huge fan of coconut, which is one of my favorite superfoods. You can sub in coconut milk for regular milk any time, and you can find commercially packaged coconut creamer and coconut yogurt. Another great alternative is to make coconut kefir or coconut ice cream using xylitol. I've included a kefir starter kit information in the Resources section on my website. Also, see page 281 for an amazing recipe for coconut ice cream that you can even enjoy in Cycle 1. Be aware, however, that this treat is *really* high in calories, so don't overdo it. A ½-cup serving counts as 2 servings of fat.

## NOT ALL MILKS ARE CREATED EQUAL

- **Soy milk.** Absolutely not. If you want to know why, turn to Chapter 4. There is *no* joy in soy!

- **Rice, almond and hemp milks.** These aren't terrible, and in a pinch, I suppose you can have a bit here and there—say, you are in a health-food restaurant and want to throw some in your coffee or tea. Generally, though, I prefer coconut milk because it has far more nutritional value. Rice and hemp milks can have a lot of sugar, and even the sugar-free versions are loaded with carbohydrates. I don't see any nutrient value to offset this, so you're way better off with my friend the coconut. However, if you really don't like or can't find coconut milk, my fallback is unsweetened almond milk.

## GETTING YOUR GOAT AND KEEPING YOUR SHEEP

Now, if you are a die-hard dairy lover, I have some very good news for you: even if you can't tolerate cow's milk, you might be okay with goat's and sheep's milk in Cycle 2. Because the fat globules don't cluster together and the protein forms a softer curd, it might be easier for you to digest. Sheep and goats are also more likely to be pasture-fed and drug-free than most commercially raised dairy cows (see the Discontented Cows on pages 100–102).

The best possible way to consume this type of milk is raw and fermented, in the form of kefir or yogurt. This gives you some amazing healthy bacteria, which serve as pre- and probiotics. But you can also have some feta cheese, some goat's or sheep's milk cheese and some goat's or sheep's milk yogurt, although these products all tend to be sharper and tangier than their cow counterparts.

For now, we're going to eliminate dairy for 21 days to give your system a chance to calm down. But you can try these dairy products in Cycle 2, when you might discover that you can have a little plain Greek-style yogurt as well.

 ## DAIRY-FREE AND LOVING IT

When I spoke with Michele after her first dairy-free week, she had already noticed an improvement in her skin. By week 2, her acne was almost gone, and by the final week of Cycle 1, her skin was glowing.

"I can't remember when my skin looked this good," she told me. "Plus, I feel like I've got way more energy, and my head is clearer. I just didn't realize how much dairy was weighing me down."

# HOW THE VIRGIN DIET WORKED FOR ME

Pamela Bruner
Age 48

Zirconia,
North Carolina

**Height:**
5'5"

**Starting Weight:**
139 pounds

**Waist:** 29"
**Hips:** 35.5"

**Current Weight:**
122 pounds

**Waist:** 26"
**Hips:** 34"

**Lost:** 17 pounds

Before I found JJ's program, I felt like I had a pretty good diet and my body was okay. I've certainly slipped a bit in the last few years, but I hadn't stepped on the scale in a long time and was shocked to see that my weight had climbed to 139. It was the first of many surprises on this program.

I remember saying to JJ, "I think I look pretty good for 48 years old." And she asked, "Why not just look good, period?" I saw that if I didn't give her program a try, I'd be settling for second best.

The first 5 days were challenging because of cravings, mostly for dairy and sugar. The rest of the items were easy for me to eliminate. However, I felt cleaner and clearer almost immediately, within a couple days. That helped me keep going.

On JJ's program, I felt like I was treating my body much better. Previously, I wasn't making sure that I fed my body high-quality protein every day, and I wasn't keeping away from sugar and other potential allergens. I was also using food far too much as a comfort mechanism.

One great thing was the weight loss was fast! I love how fast the pounds fell off.

Besides the weight, two things really stick out to me. One is my energy level. I can go all day with no drop in energy and good focus and concentration.

The other big difference is my waistline. Now my stomach is just flat and I can see my ab muscles. I feel very fit, much more than I used to.

Looking toward the future, I believe that I have true control over what I eat, and I can choose to eat a diet that makes me feel great and has food I really enjoy, too! I'm so grateful for this program.

# PLUCK THE EGGS, CORN AND PEANUTS

**6**

There are two problems with eggs, corn and peanuts. One is that they often provoke a lot of food sensitivities, so they are all three very high-FI foods. The other is that each of them is inflammatory—tending to create inflammation.

I know I've thrown a lot of health concepts at you throughout this book, but if you only remember one, inflammation is the one I want you to keep in mind. The reason the Virgin Diet works so quickly and so well is because we pull the foods that are most likely to set off inflammation. Gluten sets off inflammation by triggering leaky gut. Soy worsens inflammation by messing with your hormones and your thyroid. Dairy also messes with your hormones and is highly reactive, setting you up for leaky gut and inflammation as well.

In this chapter, we'll look at three of the most pro-inflammatory foods I know: eggs, corn and peanuts. We'll also take a closer look at inflammation itself. The fastest way to lose 7 pounds and look years younger is to pull inflammatory foods out of your diet and load up with healing foods and supplements. You've already made a terrific start, now we're going to take the process one step further.

# MAKE AN OIL CHANGE

The types of fats you eat can change the inflammatory response in your body. Raw nuts and seeds are one place to start. They're full of healthy oils and have lots of other health benefits as well. Eat them in moderation, but enjoy. Your limit is 1 to 3 servings per day, and 1 serving is 5 Brazil or Macadamia nuts; 10 walnuts, almonds or cashews; or a tablespoon of nut butter (not peanut butter).

I love palm fruit oil—it's one of my favorite superfoods—and when you get to know it, you will love it, too. It is rich in tocotrienols (members of the vitamin E family) and beta-carotene. It is a highly sustainable crop. You can heat it at high temperatures without damaging it. What's not to love?

I also love coconut oil, another rock star. It is rich in monolaurin (a great immune booster), caprylic acid (a fatty acid that fights candida) and medium-chain triglycerides (fat-burning fatty acids).

Another great choice, if you can find it, is ghee, or clarified butter, ideally from grass-fed cows. Ghee has no milk solids, so it's okay even for Cycle 1.

You can absolutely use extra-virgin olive oil in your salads and cold foods (with a name like that, how can I forbid it?), but don't cook with it at medium or high heat because it won't hold up well. Instead, use regular olive oil, palm fruit oil, coconut oil or sesame oil when you cook. The other oils I like to use in my salads are walnut and almond oil.

When flaxseed oil is exposed to the air, it goes bad, so I am not a big fan of it. I like freshly ground flaxseed meal much better because you can get some gut-healing fiber from it.

If you're using canola oil, that's fine. Just make sure that it's not genetically modified and that it's been cold-pressed. Do not heat it, no matter what the manufacturers say. Canola oil has been bred to be rich in omega-3s, which are fragile, and the last thing you want to do is expose them to heat.

 ## THE DANGERS OF A PRO-INFLAMMATORY DIET

Some foods fight inflammation. Some foods create it. Among the top pro-inflammatory culprits are foods high in arachidonic acid, especially corn, corn-fed beef and eggs. (For more about foods that fight inflammation, see the Healing Foods section on pages 178–183.)

The Virgin Diet removes the pro-inflammatory foods and adds foods that help reduce inflammation.

Now, don't worry, I'm not asking you to have zero arachidonic acid or pro-inflammatory fat in your system. In fact, you want a balance of anti-inflammatory and pro-inflammatory fats. If you have too many anti-inflammatory fats in your system, you will have blood that's really thin. If you get a cut, you could bleed excessively. But if you have too many pro-inflammatory chemicals in your body, you have thick, sticky blood and are at risk for heart disease.

As with most things in life, what you want is a nice balance—and the Virgin Diet gives you just that. It removes the more pro-inflammatory foods and adds foods that help reduce inflammation.

# LETTING GO OF EGGS

Miriam had never had a weight problem until she passed the age of 45. Then, gradually, year by year, she began to look "soft," as she put it.

"Forget the fact that I was bloated and constipated all the time," she wrote me later. "I just assumed that this was the way things were going to go for me and that menopause was responsible for my ongoing battle with low energy, intestinal discomfort and that extra weight. I assumed that my body had a mind of its own, that what was happening was out of my control and that I should just accept my new, fluffy stage of life."

Luckily, Miriam attended one of my lectures and realized that she did not have to accept her symptoms or her weight gain. Much as she hated giving up her favorite foods, she acknowledged that she had to cut at least some of the 7 high-FI foods out of her diet.

"Within a week of eliminating dairy and eggs, I felt mentally sharper and clear-headed," she wrote me. "Within 2 weeks, the gas and bloating were gone. And in about 3 weeks, I saw my weight *move down*. Within a few months, all the weight had come off. And while 13 pounds may not seem like much to some folks, to me it was huge because not only was my body fat melting, but I also looked younger and sexier. I never expected to ever look that great again!"

Like Miriam, you might not even realize that you're sensitive to eggs, even though a surprising number of people are. Do you notice gas, bloating and heartburn up to 2 days after eating eggs or foods containing eggs? Eggs have also been linked with eczema and psoriasis.

This makes me sad because eggs are a fabulous source of protein and other nutrients. I used to love them so much that I ate them every day. I think they are one of nature's perfect foods. So why do so many people have so much trouble with them?

My theory is that it may not be just the eggs themselves. It could also be what the chickens are being fed (GMO corn and soy) and the medications that they are being treated with. Remember, you are what you eat, ate. One of my clients found that she can eat eggs from her farmer's collective, where the chickens must be fed a nice, healthy diet. But if she eats any other eggs, even organic eggs from the supermarket, she gets sick. In other words, if you're eating eggs from a chicken who's fed soy and corn, and you're sensitive to soy and corn, you are going to have a problem.

## CORN-FED CHICKENS VERSUS EXCELLENT EGGS

Actually, most eggs you can buy come from chickens that were fed corn or soy, which changes their fatty acid profile. When chickens eat corn, their eggs are rich in arachidonic acid, making them more pro-inflammatory (see The Dangers of a Pro-Inflammatory Diet section on page 111).

However, a chicken that is allowed to roam free in the barnyard and eat whatever it chooses will produce an egg with a better balance of polyunsaturated fats. Barnyard eggs have 3 to 6 times the vitamin D as hen-house eggs because of the chickens' sun exposure. These barnyard eggs have higher omega-3 content as well. Their fatty acid levels also reflect the chickens' diet.

## WHERE EGGS HIDE

| | | |
|---|---|---|
| Baked goods | Flan | Meringues |
| Batter mixes | French toast | Noodles |

| | | |
|---|---|---|
| Bavarian cream | Fritters | Pancakes |
| Boiled dressing | Frosting | Puddings |
| Bouillon | Hollandaise sauce | Quiche |
| Breaded foods | Ice cream | Salad dressings |
| Breads | Macaroons | Sauces |
| Cake flours | Malted drinks | Sausages |
| Creamy fillings | Marshmallows | Soufflés |
| Custards | Mayonnaise | Tartar sauce |
| Egg drop soup | Meat loaf | Waffles |

### EGGS MAY BE LISTED ON LABELS AS:

| | | |
|---|---|---|
| Albumin | Globulin | Ovomucoid |
| Egg protein | Livetin | Ovovitellin |
| Egg white | Ovalbumin | Powdered egg |
| Egg yolk | Ovomucin | Vitellin |

Obviously, you can find eggs in omelets, quiches and other breakfast dishes. But remember that eggs are ubiquitous in baked goods, pancakes, breads and salads, including tuna and potato salads. Eggs are also frequently found in meat loaf, crab cakes, soups (think egg drop and matzo ball), crepes, zucchini fritters, stuffing, noodles and meatballs, so you will need to avoid all of these foods. Always read the ingredient lists on food labels and question your server carefully in restaurants. You'll be surprised how many foods contain eggs.

Be aware that most egg replacers do not equal the nutrient quality of real eggs. They only replace the structural quality of eggs, which means there is zero reason to eat them. You have many high-quality protein foods to choose from, such as fish, chicken and grass-fed beef. Liquid egg replacers, such as Egg Beaters, are made of egg whites and therefore should not be used as alternatives to eggs.

 ## CUT THE CORN

Corn is a pro-inflammatory food as well as a high-glycemic one, meaning that it can cause your blood sugar to spike. It's also one of our most genetically modified foods, and as we've seen, there can be a lot of issues with GMOs.

Symptoms of corn sensitivities are similar to other food intolerance reactions, including rashes and hives, migraines, joint pain, mood disorders, temporary depression, insomnia, eczema, fatigue, joint pain, hyperactivity in children, night sweats, dark circles around the eyes, repeated ear infections and urinary tract infections and a constant battle with sinus problems.

Like soy, dairy, gluten and eggs, corn is simply everywhere. Food processors use it in a variety of ways, such as cornstarch, corn syrup and corn oil. And high-fructose corn syrup is a popular sweetener used in just about everything. So you'll have to become a bit of a corn detective, hunting down corn in its many hiding places. Otherwise you'll have to stick to fresh, natural and unprocessed foods, which I personally find easier, healthier and more satisfying anyway.

# A CHEAP, UNHEALTHY GRAIN

**In just one ear of corn, you get 15 grams of insulin-spiking, inflammatory sugar.**

Many people think of corn as a vegetable, but in fact, it's a grain. It's one of the worst of all the grains because it tends to be allergenic, is high on the glycemic index and has a pro-inflammatory omega-6 fatty acid profile. As a high-glycemic starch, corn easily breaks down into sugar. In just one ear of corn, you get 15 grams of insulin-spiking, inflammatory sugar.

Yet, corn is the most abundant grain produced in America. That's because it is cheap feed for animals and an enormously profitable ingredient in high-fructose corn syrup. So what else is wrong with corn?

- **Almost all U.S. corn is genetically modified.** If you want to know more about what's wrong with GMOs, see pages 88–89. If you want to know how to avoid GMOs, see the handbook in the Resources section on my website.

- **Corn is host to 22 different types of fungi.** One of the worst is aflatoxin, a deadly and highly carcinogenic toxin that the U.S. Department of Agriculture tests for. This condemned corn supply often ends up in animal feeds, both livestock and pets. I find that frightening, don't you?

- **Corn is high in lectins.** As we've seen, they bind to your microvilli, the small fibers that extend from your intestinal walls. As a result, you can't properly absorb nutrients, your gut flora is altered and you might develop leptin resistance. You might also injure your gut lining, which can lead to leaky gut. (For more on what's wrong with lectins, see page 69.)

But probably the very worst thing about corn is its presence in high-fructose corn syrup, which I find so disturbing that I've devoted a whole section to it.

## HIGH-FRUCTOSE CORN SYRUP

Fructose is the type of sugar that is found in fruit. I am not really worried about you eating an apple, though. In fact, I am very pro-apple, pro-berry and for other types of low- and moderate-glycemic fruit.

Those are the natural foods that our bodies were meant to consume. In some processed foods, however, a high-fructose content causes what we eat to bypass our hunger response and keeps us eating even when we've had more than enough. This is especially true of foods that contain high-fructose corn syrup, a totally unnatural creation that is completely different from anything that is ideal, normal or healthy for the body.

The fructose in high-fructose corn syrup is metabolized differently than other sugars. It can elevate triglyceride levels. It can raise blood pressure. Unlike glucose, it's metabolized in the liver, where it helps favor the production of fat. And, unlike glucose, fructose doesn't stimulate insulin secretion or enhance leptin production. As we saw earlier, insulin helps regulate blood sugar, and leptin regulates appetite by signaling the body when you're full. Neither of these processes happen when you have insulin and leptin resistance going on.

However, even when you're healthy, fructose is not part of that self-regulating system. It does not signal your body that you are full, and it's absorbed far more rapidly than regular sugar. As a result, fructose can easily entice you to overeat.

High-fructose corn syrup is also bad for your intestines. High doses of free fructose can make the intestinal lining more permeable and loosen up the tight junctions that are supposed to keep partially digested food from leaking out into your system. As explained in Chapter 1, this creates leaky gut and triggers your immune system, creating new food sensitivities, inflammation and a host of painful symptoms. In other words, you may have a new cycle going on:

High-fructose corn syrup → damages gut integrity →
creates leaky gut → sets you up for more sensitivity →
creates inflammation → You gain weight that you cannot lose.

## PLUCK THE PESTICIDES, TOO

Here's another reason to cut the corn: genetically modified crops are built to withstand large amounts of pesticides. We have 80 million acres of corn in the United States, so that's a lot of poison going into the ecosystem.

> Genetically modified crops are built to withstand large amounts of pesticides.

The runoff from these crops has to go somewhere. In the Midwestern corn belt, the runoff flows into the Mississippi River and then into the Gulf of Mexico, where it has already killed off marine life in a 12,000-square-mile area. Do you want to be part of that?

## EATING WHAT YOU ATE, ATE

Even if you're not eating corn, you might be eating corn-fed beef or chicken. Most commercially produced beef and chicken falls into that category because it fattens up livestock fast. In fact, farmers call it "the swine-fattening formula." So, when you eat meat or chicken, you are ultimately probably still consuming corn, and genetically modified corn at that. This is why I want you to avoid anything other than grass-fed beef and have a good relationship with your farmers and butchers so you know what the foods you eat were eating.

## CORN-FED VERSUS GRASS-FED BEEF

I'm a huge fan of grass-fed beef. It is harder to find and more expensive than corn-fed beef, but grass-fed beef is better for human health in a dozen different ways.

For example, a study by the U.S. Department of Agriculture and researchers at Clemson University in South Carolina in 2009 found that compared with grain-fed beef, grass-fed beef was lower in total fat; higher in beta-carotene; higher in vitamin E; higher in the B vitamins thiamin and riboflavin; and higher in calcium, magnesium and potassium.

We also know that grass-fed beef is 2 to 3 times higher in anti-inflammatory omega-3s, plus it is lower in calories and leaner. As we saw in the previous chapter, it's also higher in the amazing fatty acid CLA, which helps burn fat. Additionally, grass-fed beef is lower in saturated fat. I am happy to call grass-fed beef a clean, lean protein and give it a place in the Virgin Diet.

## SORRY, POPCORN IS *NOT* A HEALTHY SNACK

There's a popular myth going around that popcorn is a healthy, low-cal snack. That is *not* true, but this is:

- Popcorn is generally made with damaged fats.

- Microwave popcorn may have toxins in the bag liners.

- Popcorn is high-glycemic (makes your blood sugar spike, setting up problems with hunger, leptin resistance and insulin resistance).

- Popcorn is a trigger food: it makes you want more salt, starch and fat.

## WHERE CORN HIDES

| | | |
|---|---|---|
| Breakfast cereals | Glucose | Margarine |
| Cerelose | Grits | Popcorn |
| Corn chips | Hominy | Puretose |
| Dextrose | Maize | Sweetose |
| Dyno | | Vegetable oil |

# PASS ON THE PEANUTS

Another supposedly healthy snack is peanuts. Although peanuts may not be as detrimental as some of the other 7 foods to avoid, they are one of the more potentially reactive foods, and there are far better options out there in the tree nut family. (Peanuts aren't actually nuts, they are legumes!)

Why am I so antipeanut? Peanuts have a high risk for aflatoxin mold, which is toxic and provokes a lot of allergies. Other legumes offer more nutrients per calorie (think black beans, white beans, kidney beans, etc.), and tree nuts have a far superior fatty acid profile. Plus, most of the peanut butters out there have added sugar (so kids will like them) and added fat (often trans fat, the worst kind) to make it smooth.

Peanuts tend to trigger outright food allergies and IgE reactions—the immediate, severe, acute and potentially deadly allergic reactions. We are also seeing more IgG (the slower, food-sensitivity response) reactions with peanuts.

Peanut oil may be atherogenic, which means it may cause arterial plaque to form.

Peanuts are also high in phytic acid and lectins, which as we've seen, is not so good for the gut. Basically, you don't miss anything by letting this food go. Where you'd normally eat peanuts, try raw or slow-roasted tree nuts (walnuts, almonds, cashews, macadamia nuts or pecans), and where you'd normally have peanut butter, try tree nut butter (cashew, almond, macadamia or pecan—just make sure it's sugar-free). This is one of those lateral shifts that you're going to find you like so much better that you won't miss peanuts at all.

## WHERE PEANUTS AND PEANUT OIL HIDE

| | |
|---|---|
| Baked goods | Ice cream |
| Baking mixes | Margarine |
| Battered foods | Marzipan |
| Biscuits | Milk formula |
| Breakfast cereals | Pastry |
| Candy | Peanut butter |
| Cereal-based products | Satay sauce and dishes |
| Chili sauce | Soups |
| Chinese dishes | Thai dishes |
| Cookies | Vegetable fat |
| Egg rolls | Vegetable oil |

## PEANUTS MAY BE LISTED ON LABELS AS:

| | |
|---|---|
| Emulsifier (uncommon) | Oriental sauce |
| Flavoring | Peanut |
| Ground nut | Peanut butter |

# HOW THE VIRGIN DIET WORKED FOR ME

Laureen Shefchik
Age 49

Union,
Kentucky

**Height:**
5'2"

**Starting Weight:**
229 pounds

**Waist:** 43"
**Hips:** 47"

**Current Weight:**
179 pounds

**Waist:** 34"
**Hips:** 43"

**Lost:** 50 pounds

I've been on JJ's plan for 1 year now. It has been a wonderful, life-changing experience.

Over the past 30 years, I have lost and gained a few hundred pounds. One year ago, all I felt was frustration, depression, fatigue and overall "overwhelm." I was thinking seriously of having a surgical procedure to help me lose weight.

Then I got an email about JJ's plan. After reading the details of the program, tears slowly trickled down my cheeks. This sounded like a new beginning for me. On October 4, 2010, I recorded my weight at 229 lbs. I wore a size 2X, or 20/22 women's. Yet, my family and I had been eating organic food and a pretty healthy diet for about 10 years. I cook and bake from scratch and don't eat processed foods. We haven't eaten MSG, soy or high-fructose corn syrup in years.

JJ took gluten, peanuts, dairy and eggs out of my diet, on top of soy, which I'd already removed. I could not believe the results. In the first 14 days, I began to have more energy than I have had in years! My brain fog was lifting, and I felt light—not so heavy or depressed. I had suffered from sinus problems, headaches, infections and other symptoms. These symptoms became much less severe, and my headaches disappeared completely—a direct result of pulling out the dairy.

After 28 days on JJ's plan, I had lost almost 14 pounds and felt like a new woman. Now, 1 year later, I have lost 50 pounds, and I wear size 12/14! I will continue to reach for my body's perfect weight.

I have people ask me every day, "What are you doing? You look fabulous!!!" I always feel so grateful to JJ for giving me a life that's worth living again!

My client Lisa was able to stick to her diet and exercise plan all day, but at night her discipline dissolved. As soon as she started to relax, her sugar cravings would kick in, and Lisa would hunt down all the sweet treats in the house like a junkie seeking her next fix. Once, she even stole her kids' Halloween candy.

"I'm ashamed of myself," she told me, "but I can't stop."

Now as it turns out, this is more than just an issue of poor willpower. In fact, I don't believe in willpower at all. This was a situation in which Lisa's genetics were making things tough for her because those big sugar cravings were partly due to her genes. As it turns out, our tastes are genetically determined to a large extent: some of us will like bitter, sour or sweet more than others. Lisa truly had been born with a sweet tooth.

> Our tastes are genetically determined to a large extent.

Plus, Lisa had a second issue that was exacerbating that sweet tooth: she struggled with chronic stress because of poor sleep, young kids and a demanding job. This stress was depleting her serotonin levels, which also made her crave the carbs. So Lisa's genetics plus her life circumstances had created a very challenging situation.

Lisa's evening sugar consumption led to multiple problems: mood swings, blood sugar crashes, food cravings and sugar addiction. In effect, poor Lisa had become a sugar hostage to her out-of-balance blood sugar and her genetic sweet tooth. So, we had to pull her off the sugar and feed her sweet tooth in other ways. We replaced her evening sugar binge with a hot bath and a great book, and we gave her some healthy, sweet-tasting foods earlier in the day to satisfy her sweet tooth without triggering her cravings.

The good news is that when Lisa saw how sugar was sabotaging her weight loss, her mood and her health, she was motivated to dump it. Let me share with you what I shared with her.

 ## SUGAR WOES

We are eating more sugar than ever. We eat 140 pounds of sugar a year, but 10,000 years ago, we ate only 22 teaspoons a year.

This is just not good for us. Period.

**We eat 140 pounds of sugar a year.**

Look, I really get how good sugar tastes, but it doesn't just contain empty calories. It is a secret saboteur that undermines your weight-loss efforts in a number of different ways:

- Sugar puts you on a blood sugar roller coaster, where your hunger spikes and crashes.
- Sugar disrupts your insulin metabolism.
- Sugar raises your stress hormones, which raises the set point to burn off fat.
- Sugar feeds yeast, which contributes to yeast overgrowth and sugar cravings.
- Sugar feeds bad bacteria, which cause your body to extract more calories from the food you eat, store them as fat and create digestive problems, including gas and bloating.

- Sugar dampens your immune system, which sets you up for more food intolerance.
- Sugar makes you better at storing fat.
- Sugar creates more cravings: when you eat sweet, you crave sweet.
- Sugar depletes nutrients.

That's a long, ugly list, but I believe in knowing your enemy. So let's take a closer look.

 ## STRESS IS NOT SWEET

Did you know that stress can actually raise your blood sugar? Fasting blood sugar is the measure of how high your blood sugar is after you haven't eaten for at least 8 hours. It's used to estimate your risk of diabetes. I have often seen clients with a good diet who are eating well and exercising, but if they are under chronic stress, they have a higher fasting blood sugar.

> Did you know that stress can actually raise your blood sugar?

Higher fasting blood sugar leads to higher insulin, which creates inflammation. Inflammation reinforces insulin resistance and leptin resistance. (Leptin is the hormone that regulates feelings of hunger and fullness, so if you have leptin resistance, you are likely to keep eating even after you're full.)

Stress also makes you crave sugar. That's because stress lowers serotonin, the feel-good chemical that helps you fight depression, sleep well, avoid headaches and generally experience optimism, self-confidence and strong self-esteem. It also lowers dopamine, the pleasure chemical that accompanies excitement. So when you're under stress, you crave both sugar (to replenish your serotonin) and overall calories (to rev up your dopamine).

> When you're under stress, you crave both sugar and overall calories.

As a result, stress sets you off on a blood sugar roller coaster. You wake up tired and stressed, so you grab a big caffeinated drink and a large, sugary treat—maybe a muffin or a toaster pastry. Your blood sugar comes up, and insulin surges to bring it back down. Often, the insulin overcorrects, especially if you're insulin resistant. So your body pumps out too much insulin, and your blood sugar drops again. Now it's the middle of the morning, and you are wondering, *Where's my second cup of coffee and my second muffin?*

This isn't good for your weight loss, your inflammation level, your mood or your stress levels because all that caffeine and sugar is not exactly calming you down. Plus, eating too many refined carbohydrates raises your levels of triglycerides and LDL (low-density lipoprotein, the bad cholesterol), putting you at risk of heart disease, hardening of the arteries and stroke.

# THE GLYCEMIC INDEX

Glucose is the main fuel source for your brain, and you want a slowly released, steady supply of it. The glycemic index is a rating system developed to measure how the food you eat affects your blood sugar levels. Glucose is set at 100, and all other foods are measured accordingly. The higher its glycemic index rating, the greater effect a food will have on your blood sugar. Meanwhile, foods that are lower on the glycemic index are generally less refined and have more fiber, giving you a nice, slow release of energy. So, the best choice to keep your blood sugar balanced is to stick to low-glycemic foods.

Now, I should tell you that the glycemic index remains controversial. Some people claim that it has no clinical significance, whereas others have written entire books recommending we eat according to this rating system. I think it is useful, but within limits. The important thing to remember is that it is just one tool for understanding nutrition and is not the end-all.

For example, there are some foods that are healthy but have a high-glycemic index, such as beets and carrots. And there are foods that are low on the glycemic index that aren't always healthy. For example, fructose—one of the types of sugar found in fruit, vegetables and some grains—is low on the glycemic index scale, yet we know it is the sugar most likely to cause arterial plaque and can also lead to insulin resistance. Milk is also low on the glycemic index, but it too can lead to insulin resistance (see Chapter 5, "Dump the Dairy").

Another issue with the glycemic index is quantity. Beets and carrots may be high on the index, but you can only eat so many of them. Potatoes are also high on the glycemic index (although they are basically just big lumps of sugar), but unlike beets and carrots, you usually don't eat just a tablespoon or two of them. Usually, you're having a whole potato.

I think the glycemic index points you in two very useful directions: *eat real foods, rather than processed ones,* and *consume a lot of fiber.* That's why I focus on low-glycemic, high-fiber carbs in the Virgin Diet. They'll be way better for giving you a nice, steady supply of energy than high-glycemic items, like potatoes, or low-fiber items, such as juice.

## YOUR GLYCEMIC LOAD

A concept that is probably more useful than the glycemic index is the glycemic load, a concept that tells us more about how a carbohydrate actually affects your blood sugar. The glycemic load is the glycemic index multiplied by the amount of carbohydrates that is actually being consumed.

Remember how I said we eat just a few bites of carrot but a whole potato? Well, a single carrot has a glycemic index of 131 and contains only 4 grams of carbs, so its glycemic load is (1.31 x 4), or about 5. One mashed potato has a glycemic index of 104 and 37 grams of carbohydrates, so its glycemic load is (1.04 x 37), or just over 38.

In fact, recent research reveals that our health is not as much affected by the glycemic index of a single meal or snack as it is by the cumulative impact of the glycemic load we consume throughout the day. This is why 1 serving of roasted beets or a few baby carrots are fine, but a big glass of carrot or beet juice is not. The glycemic index doesn't tell you the whole story. You have to look at the glycemic load.

## SUPPLEMENTS TO HELP BALANCE YOUR BLOOD SUGAR

So, what's the best way to solve the sugar problem? Balance your blood sugar.

Following the Virgin Diet is going to help you with that. Eating regular, correctly sized portions of clean, lean protein; healthy fats; and low-glycemic, high-fiber carbs is the perfect recipe for balanced blood sugar because the protein, fats and fiber keep the carbs from pushing up your blood sugar too quickly, and the carbs are mainly low-glycemic to begin with. (See "The Glycemic Index" and "Your Glycemic Load" on pages 128–130.)

You can also use supplements to help balance your blood sugar. The four horsemen for blood sugar balance are chromium, magnesium, vanadium and zinc. You want to take a good multivitamin and mineral formula with these or take a good blood sugar balancing formula that contains these nutrients. I like to have people take extra chromium—about 500 micrograms 3 times per day, for a total of 1,000 to 2,000 micrograms per day. You can also take berberine, a "two for one" supplement that both balances blood sugar and fights microbes in the gastrointestinal tract.

Finally, make sure you're getting enough vitamin D. Have your doctor run a 25-hydroxy vitamin D test to see where your levels are (see pages 68–69 for more information). You should be in the 60 to 80 ng/ml range, and you need to watch this throughout the year. Vitamin D will vary depending on where you live and if you're using sunscreen. Some people genetically have lower vitamin D levels. I find that most people need to supplement at least 2,000 IU to 5,000 IU per day on an ongoing basis. If your levels are low, you should take up to 10,000 IU per day until you reach ideal levels. You want to make sure that you're taking vitamin D3—because that's the kind your body makes and uses.

Here's another supplement I love for combating sugar and carb cravings, 5-HTP, which stands for 5-hydroxytryptophan. This amazing amino acid is well absorbed and can cross the blood–brain barrier, where it is converted to serotonin. People who are overweight tend to have lower levels of serotonin because insulin resistance can keep serotonin from reaching their brains. Two separate studies of obese women have shown that the women experienced weight loss, reduced appetite and reduced carbohydrate intake when they were given 5-HTP.[17, 18] I recommend 100 to 300 milligrams 1 to 3 times per day.

Another great two for one is glutamine, my number one gut healer, which can also help with sugar and alcohol cravings. Alpha-lipoic acid is also amazing, both for improving insulin sensitivity and for healing the liver, which will help you metabolize fat better.

Finally, don't forget your fiber! Fiber will slow the release of glucose into your blood, keeping those levels nice and steady, just the way we like them.

## TAPERING OFF

If you've been eating a high-carb, high-sugar diet, the easiest way to switch over without crashing and burning is to taper off by using fruit. The first week of Cycle 1, have 2 extra servings of low- to moderate-glycemic fruits. The next week, go down to 1 extra serving. By week 3, you should be fine.

 ## PROTEIN PACKS A PUNCH

Another thing to help with sugar cravings is to get the right portions of clean, lean protein 3 times per day. You also need to make sure you're digesting the protein you consume. I find that people are often eating their protein without properly digesting it, either because they're drinking too much water with their meal or because they lack digestive enzymes.

The easiest way to check your stomach acid levels is to do a trial of digestive enzymes that contain betaine HCL and pepsin. Unless you have a history of ulcers, you can do this type of trial to see if the enzymes help you feel better. If you feel uncomfortably full for a long time after you eat, suffer from acid reflux, routinely burp after a meal or suffer from rosacea, those are even stronger signs that you would probably benefit from enzymes. Your stomach acid lowers as you age and because of stress, so you should also consider an enzyme trial if you are over the age of 30 or under chronic stress.

Start with one enzyme taken with a meal and raise the dose by one with each meal until you feel the mildest warm sensation in your chest. Then, reduce your dose by one capsule: that is your standard dose to take with each meal. As you are healing your gut and handling your stress better, you may notice that you need less, so if you notice that mild warmth again, reduce your dosage further.

##  FASTING INSULIN AND GLUCOSE

As part of your regular checkup, your doctor routinely tests your fasting blood sugar. You want that to be in the 70 to 80 milligrams range. When your fasting insulin is tested, it should be in the range of 2 to 5. You also want to be tested for hemoglobin A1c, which is a marker of what's been going on over the last 3 to 4 months with your blood sugar. Has it been riding high too much of the time? Has it been at a normal level? You ideally want a number of 5.0 or less, but at least under 5.5. Remember, you are not striving for normal or "in range" here, you are striving for optimal numbers because that will help you achieve optimal health.

# DON'T BLAME THE SWEET TOOTH

Now at this point, you might be freaking out and thinking, *I like sweet! Don't blame me. It's not my fault. I have a sweet tooth.*

If you have a sweet tooth, I agree: it's not your fault. If you have had a sweet tooth all of your life, you can bet that it is probably in your genes. I don't think you should battle your genes. You should work with them. So if you have a genetic sweet tooth, I will be sympathetic to you. I get it.

However, having a genetic sweet tooth does *not* mean that you have to eat cookies. Don't try that one with me. It won't fly. You've got two other choices and I'll help you with both of them. My top choice is to retrain your taste buds. Learn to appreciate raspberries, strawberries and blueberries. Cinnamon, vanilla, cloves and almonds can also feed that sweet tooth once you learn to savor their natural sweetness.

> Having a sweet tooth does *not* mean that you have to eat cookies.

Here's your second choice: dark chocolate. Yes, you heard me. The nutritionist is telling you to eat chocolate. But only 1 to 2 ounces per day, only if it's dark—and only if you can stick to that amount. You should look for organic dark chocolate at 70 percent cacao or above: the higher the cacao percentage, the better. If you have 2 ounces, count it as a high-fiber carb serving and adjust accordingly. Now remember, Cycle 1 is where we really buckle down and yank the sugar, so leave out the dark chocolate during Cycle 1.

Okay, I have a confession to make. I personally cannot bring dark chocolate into the house. I don't have a sweet tooth, but if I bring home dark chocolate, I eat every bit of it. I have to buy a small bar and share it with a friend or toss out the extra so I get only my allotted 2 ounces.

# IF YOU HAVE A SWEET TOOTH...

- Mix chocolate vegan pea-rice protein powder with a little coconut milk and cinnamon, which is a nice blood sugar balancer. Add some decaf or regular coffee powder for an amazing hot or iced mocha.

- Mix a little bit of coconut milk with some chocolate protein powder to make a sauce. Add berries and top with chopped almonds. Mmmm...

- Make your own nutella by mixing almond butter with slightly liquefied chocolate protein powder (liquefy by adding a tiny amount of coconut milk or water). Then, add cinnamon. A tablespoon of this is 1 serving—then put it *away!*

- Smear some almond butter onto apple slices and sprinkle with cinnamon.

- Roast a sweet potato and add some cinnamon and chopped walnuts.

- Vanilla naturally raises your serotonin as soon as you smell it, so add some vanilla to your coffee or to anything you're making with coconut milk.

- Nutmeg and cloves help satisfy a sweet tooth, and they go great with orange foods like carrots, sweet potatoes, pumpkin and butternut squash.

## THE MYTH OF "HEALTHY SUGARS"

I hate to break it to you, but the idea of healthy sugars is crazy. I'm sorry. They don't exist.

Some people argue that agave and honey are natural. Agave is higher in fructose than high-fructose corn syrup. Read on for the problems with fructose. Natural or not, it could not be worse for you.

Honey, however, could have some homeopathic benefits for allergies. If you have immune responses to bits of mold and dust, organic honey can strengthen your immune system and help you handle those things better. This needs to be locally grown organic raw honey, and you only need about a half-teaspoon a day.

> The idea of healthy sugars is crazy.

## FRUCTOSE: THE WORST SUGAR OF THEM ALL

Not all sugars are created equal. Fructose, which is one of the sugars found in fruits and vegetables, is much, much worse. You don't need to worry about the fructose found in whole fruits and vegetables that you consume. The problem is when you start drinking juice or consuming high-fructose corn syrup or agave-sweetened "health foods," because that approach gives you super-high levels of fructose, which set you up for weight gain and other health risks. One study estimated that high-fructose corn syrup accounts for as much as 40 percent of caloric sweeteners used in the United States. The study looked at both short- and long-term effects of high-fructose corn syrup on body weight, body fat and triglycerides in rats. The rats were fed different chows: one with high-fructose corn syrup, one with sucrose and one regular one. In both the short term and long term, the rats fed the high-fructose corn syrup chow gained more overall weight and fat around their waists and had higher triglycerides than either the control rats or the rats who ate the chow with sucrose. These results suggest that excessive consumption of high-fructose corn syrup may contribute to the incidence of obesity in humans.[19]

An overabundance of fructose first found its way into our diets when we learned how to genetically modify corn. As a result, it became very cheap to produce high-fructose corn syrup, a sweetener and preservative that is in just about every processed food you can think of, not to mention one of the main ingredients in full-sugar sodas.

What's wrong with fructose? Where do I start?

Fructose can exacerbate high blood pressure. In fact, researchers use fructose on lab rats if they need them to become hypertensive for a study. Fructose can also elevate uric acid, which can cause gout. Fructose can also cause small bacterial intestinal overgrowth, intestinal yeast overgrowth, insulin resistance and kidney disease. Fructose can poke holes in your small intestine creating leaky gut.

Would you believe me if I told you that these are the *least* bad things it does?

The biggest problem with fructose is that it has a low-glycemic index, meaning that it doesn't raise your blood sugar. That's because fructose is metabolized differently from glucose. Fructose doesn't trigger your brain to release leptin (the fullness hormone), which means that you can consume an enormous amount of fructose calories without your brain ever realizing that you are full. Yet, because you're loading your body up with calories, your blood sugar spins out of control, and you develop leptin resistance. Meanwhile, 100 percent of the fructose you consume goes straight to your liver, which stores a lot of it as fat and converts the rest into free fatty acids, triglycerides and cholesterol, which turn into fat and artery-clogging plaques.

Remember back in Chapter 1 when I told you that counting calories is not the point? Here is part of what I meant: according to Dr. Robert Lustig, a professor of pediatrics in the Division of Endocrinology at the University of California, San Francisco, one-third of fructose calories ends up getting stored as fat. If you consume 120 calories of glucose, only 1 calorie is stored as fat. If you consume 120 calories of fructose, 40 calories are stored as fat. So fructose is 40 times more likely than any other sugar to make you fat—not to mention that it doesn't trigger the hormone that lets you know you are full. What I want you to imagine is that if you are eating large quantities of fructose, you are making fat.

> Fructose is 40 times more likely than any other sugar to make you fat.

Fructose just frustrates your weight-loss efforts everywhere you turn. It can also affect your fat-burning abilities after exercise, which is exactly when they should be cranked up! One study compared two groups of adults after exercise by measuring their fatty acid oxidation (i.e., fat burning). One group consumed a drink with 50 grams of glucose, and the other group consumed a drink with 50 grams of fructose. The fructose group showed 39 percent less fat oxidation after exercise as compared with the glucose group—and remember, they were consuming the same amount of calories.[20]

So, there are two morals to this story: avoid any product containing high-fructose corn syrup like the plague (see pages 117–118 for more information) and junk the juice. These products are not just extra calories. They are a type of calorie that is metabolized differently from broccoli, French fries or even a teaspoonful of white, refined sugar. The glucose in broccoli, potatoes and sugar does not all go straight to your liver. The fructose in corn syrup and fruit juice does. These calories are on a fast track to turn into fat. Not a pretty picture.

## JUNK THE JUICE

I know that fruit juices, especially fresh-squeezed, sound healthy, but I'm sorry, they are actually one of the worst weight-loss traps you can stumble into. Liquid sugars drive up your blood sugar even faster than solid sweets, and therefore your insulin goes up faster, too. Because juices are high in fructose and low in fiber, they don't have the satiety effect, which means you don't feel full. You wouldn't sit down and eat four oranges but you could easily drink the equivalent in one quick glass of juice. So you've consumed a lot of sugars that don't satisfy you. What kind of sense does that make?

You don't want drinks whose names contain the words *nectar* or *cocktail*. Both of those terms are code for "we added even more sugar." Also, avoid any product with the word *light* on it because that only means they added water and artificial sweeteners.

## FRUITS AND FRUCTOSE

Now let's get one thing straight: fruit is fabulous if you're eating the right kinds in the right amounts. I want you to choose a high-fiber, low-glycemic fruit (see page 167 to find out which fruits are low-, moderate- and high-glycemic). Berries are the best. They have so many wonderful benefits that they are one of the superfoods.

Fruit is one of the big ways that we raise our level of triglycerides, and triglycerides are how we store unused calories as fat.

One to two pieces of low- or moderate-glycemic index fruit per day should be it. And if you have issues with insulin resistance or high triglycerides, you should only have one fruit per day or maybe even none.

## WHERE SUGAR HIDES

When you're looking at labels, it can be like reading a foreign language. Let me help: all of the following mean sugar, and that means put the package down.

| | | |
|---|---|---|
| Barley malt | Date sugar | Invert sugar |
| Beet sugar | Demerara sugar | Lactose |
| Blackstrap molasses | Dextrin | Malt syrup |
| Brown sugar | Dextrose | Maltodextrin |
| Cane juice crystals | Diastatic malt | Maltose |
| Cane sugar | Diatase | Maple syrup |
| Caramel | Evaporated cane juice | Molasses |
| Carob syrup | Fructose | Raw sugar |
| Castor sugar | Fruit juice concentrate | Rice syrup |
| Confectioner's sugar | Galactose | Sucrose |
| Corn sweeteners | Glucose | Syrup |
| Corn syrup | High-fructose corn syrup | Treacle |
| D-mannose | Honey | Turbinado sugar |

# WHAT ABOUT ARTIFICIAL SWEETENERS?

Sorry, folks. These are not the solution. I believe they raise insulin. It's still a question mark, but a few studies have shown that they do. One study showed that people's bodies' began releasing insulin when they swished and spit out either sucrose or saccharine, so the insulin response started in the mouth without the subjects even having to swallow.[21] Another study showed that the effect of acesulfame K (an artificial sweetener) on insulin secretion was similar to that observed by injecting or infusing the same doses of glucose.[22] As we've just seen, when you raise your insulin level, you are telling your body to store fat. You can't access stored fat for fuel. You will be hungrier. You create insulin resistance and leptin resistance, which makes you hungrier. That makes it much more difficult to lose weight.

Plus, artificial sweeteners might cause a phenomenon called calorie disregulation. This means that your body loses the ability to correlate the degree of a food's sweetness to the amount of calories it contains. When you eat something supersweet, your body is supposed to say, "Wow! I just had a lot of calories!" Then you're satisfied after a small amount. But artificial sweeteners teach your body not to respond this way. Because your body has lost its own sense of how many calories it's consuming, you end up ingesting way more sweets than you otherwise would. A study found that "dietary factors that degrade the relationship between sweet tastes, food viscosity and calories may contribute to overeating and weight gain."[23]

Furthermore, many artificial sweeteners can be neurotoxic. That's a fancy way of saying that they deplete some of the brain chemicals that we need to lose weight. For example, many artificial sweeteners lower our levels of serotonin, the feel-good brain chemical that combats depression, helps you sleep well and generally boosts mood and well-being.[24]

Then, in the ultimate vicious cycle, low levels of serotonin make you crave more sweets!

Artificial sweeteners can also be neuroexcitatory, making it difficult to sleep and creating anxiety. And what do many of us crave when we're anxious? Sweet, starchy foods.

Even more alarming, did you know that aspartame turns into formaldehyde when it's raised over a certain temperature? Some artificial sweeteners have been found to disrupt healthy gut flora, allowing for the bad bacteria to take over, creating small intestine bacteria overgrowth, which we learned about in Chapter 1. So your apparently harmless sugar substitute might be setting you up for some serious digestive problems, which in turn will lead to weight gain.

Finally, and probably most serious of all, artificial sweeteners, like sugar, can go through a process called glycation. This is the fastest way to age your body, and it is reason enough to avoid all artificial sweeteners.

## YOUR SWEETEST OPTIONS

If you must sweeten your food, I'll allow the sugar alcohol xylitol and the sweet herb stevia. I prefer that you use xylitol or a blend of xylitol and stevia. I worry that if you use straight stevia, it might cause calorie disregulation. So I like to mix the two of them.

Xylitol can actually help you lose weight. It is a sugar alcohol, not to be confused with either alcohol or sugar. Sugar alcohols have less calories per gram than regular sugar and don't significantly raise blood

---
**Xylitol can actually help you lose weight.**

---

sugar. Xylitol specifically has some benefits not seen in other sugar alcohols. It slows down stomach emptying and suppresses ghrelin, a hormone that triggers hunger. It doesn't feed yeast, it's antibacterial, it doesn't promote cavities and it helps with bone remodeling. It is amazing stuff! It is a nutritive sweetener, if you can imagine that, making it my favorite to recommend.

## RETRAIN YOUR TASTE BUDS

If you're used to the overstimulation of diet sodas and sugar-free treats, how can you appreciate the subtle taste of berries, almonds or cinnamon? These other foods could potentially satisfy a sweet tooth, but only one that hasn't been overstimulated by the supersweetness of aspartame or sucralose. Let go of the artificial stuff and let Mother Nature show you just how sweet she can be.

## DUMP THE DIET SODAS

Even if a diet soda has zero calories, it is a nightmare in so many different ways. Besides the problems with artificial sweeteners, the phosphoric acid in sodas can actually leach the calcium from your bones. Switch to water, please. Squeeze in some lemon or lime or throw in some cucumbers or maybe a packet of Emergen-C lite. Your bones will be happier, and so will you.

But the real reason to dump the diet soda is that it could actually cause you to *gain* weight. Findings from 8 years of data collected by Sharon Fowler, MPH, and her colleagues at the University of Texas Health Science Center, San Antonio, were presented at the 2005 American Diabetes Association meeting. Fowler was quoted on WebMD: "What was surprising was when we looked at people only drinking diet soft drinks, their risk of obesity was even higher" than those drinking regular sodas. She added, "There was a 41 percent increase in risk of being overweight for every can or bottle of diet soft drink a person consumes each day." In fact, she and her colleagues found that there was more of a risk of gaining weight from drinking diet soda than from regular soda.[25] I think you get the message.

## WHERE ARTIFICIAL SWEETENERS HIDE

Sugar is not the only sweetener that goes by many names. If you see a label that includes any item on this list, put the food down and find something that has not been artificially sweetened.

| | |
|---|---|
| Acesulfame potassium | NutraSweet |
| Alitame | Saccharin |
| Aspartame | Splenda |
| Aspartame-acesulfame salt | Sucralose |
| Cyclamate | |

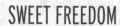

## SWEET FREEDOM

Lisa was thrilled with her weight loss, but she was even more delighted to finally feel that she had let go of her sugar cravings. Yes, sometimes she still wanted to eat sweet things, but the berries, dark chocolate and almonds she snacked on didn't set up the same round of craving, bingeing and frustration that she had experienced when she indulged in candy bars and baked goods.

"I never thought I wouldn't miss dessert," Lisa told me, "but I actually don't. I still loooooove my dark chocolate, and if I didn't have a square of *that* every night, I would definitely miss it. But that's it, you know? I have it, it tastes delicious, and then I'm satisfied." She sighed happily and added, "It's a good feeling."

Drew Matich
Age 48

Glendale,
California

**Height:**
6'4"

**Starting Weight:**
240 pounds

**Waist:** 38"

**Current Weight:**
210 pounds

**Waist:** 34"

**Lost:** 30 pounds

# HOW THE VIRGIN DIET WORKED FOR ME

Before JJ, I could eat sugar, carbs, dairy and gluten with the worst of 'em. Sure, I ate my veggies and protein, but I also put some au gratin or garlic mashed potatoes on the side. Over time I became unhappy with my weight and fat level. And more important, I was feeling less energetic and more anxious. Getting only 4 to 6 hours of nightly sleep was taking a huge toll on my endurance and motivation level at work.

Then I discovered the Virgin Diet.

The first thing that sparked my interest in JJ's approach was how commonsense it all seemed. In spite of what I would have to eliminate, I could retain a lot of what I had already been eating. In addition to replacing a meal with a Virgin Diet Shake, I tossed out the gluten, dairy and sugar. Cold turkey. I started journaling. I concentrated on eating the right veggies and proteins. And

I learned about healthy fats. An apple with a tablespoon of almond butter became my dessert staple.

Thinking back on it, I see two aspects of JJ's approach as key to my success: the one-a-day Virgin Diet Shake to replace 1 meal and the journaling. Even though there was no sugar in the smoothies, they satisfied that craving in a very healthy way. And the journaling helped me stay on task by making me accountable for everything I ate.

Obviously, I loved the result. I don't even have chocolate cravings anymore. JJ's approach gives me two things I can depend on: I know that it works for me, and I know that I can do it. Now I'm doing it for life.

# THREE CYCLES TO LOSE WEIGHT FOR GOOD

So now you're ready to begin 21 days of the Virgin Diet. Congratulations! The commitment you're making to your health and well-being is enormous. Your rewards will be enormous, too.

## 7 STEPS TO LOSING 7 POUNDS IN 7 DAYS

Just follow these 7 steps to losing 7 pounds in 7 days:

1. **Drop the top 7 high-FI foods.** For 21 days, let go of the foods that are most likely to cause food intolerance, inflammation and unbalanced blood sugar.

2. **Eat from the Virgin Diet Plate.** Assemble your meals from clean, lean proteins; healthy fats; high-fiber, low-glycemic carbs; and nonstarchy vegetables.

3. **Drink Virgin Diet Shakes.** Replace 1 or 2 meals per day with my shakes, which will help restore your digestive system and repair the damage done by the high-FI foods.

4. **Follow the golden rules of meal timing.** Eat every 4 to 6 hours. Make sure you eat within an hour of waking up and don't eat anything for the last 2 to 3 hours before bed.

5. **Stay hydrated.** Follow my Virgin Diet water guidelines.

6. **Load up on healing foods.** They'll satisfy your hunger while healing your body.

7. **Eat plenty of fabulous fiber.** Fiber will satisfy your hunger, lower your cholesterol and streamline your digestion.

In this chapter, I give you the 7 steps to losing up to 7 pounds in 7 days. I also tell you everything else you need to know about eating and drinking on the Virgin Diet. In Chapter 11, I share with you The Ultimate Meal Assembly Guide, along with my favorite meal assemblies. And in Chapter 12, I include plenty of delicious (and easy to make) recipes to get you started.

Reading your way through these chapters might seem a bit overwhelming, and at times you might find yourself wishing for a weekly plan where I just walk you through each meal. I don't want you to depend on me, however, and I don't want to tie you down either. I want you to start assembling your own meals out of optimal foods because that's what I want you to be doing for the rest of your life. This method works for my celebrity clients and for the thousands of students I've had in my weight-loss boot camps. I know it can work for you, too, so let's get started.

## STEP 1: DROP THE TOP 7 HIGH-FI FOODS

For 21 days, let go of the foods that are most likely to cause food intolerance, inflammation and unbalanced blood sugar:

| | | |
|---|---|---|
| Corn | Eggs | Peanuts |
| Dairy | Gluten | Soy |
| Sugar and artificial sweeteners | | |

## STEP 2: EAT FROM THE VIRGIN DIET PLATE

Use the Virgin Diet Plate to assemble your meals.

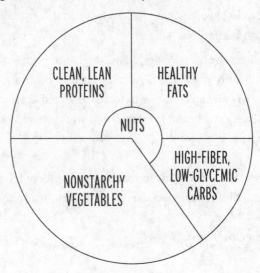

As you can see, the Virgin Diet Plate is made up of the following elements:

I want to teach
you to live by
the plate.

- Clean, lean proteins
- Healthy fats
- Nuts
- High-fiber, low-glycemic carbs
- Nonstarchy vegetables

I want to teach you to live by the plate. You start each meal with protein, healthy fats, lots of fiber and some slow low carbs, which gives you steady, sustained energy, helps you focus and turns your body into a fat-burning machine.

- The protein works with the fiber to slow down stomach emptying. That improves satiety.

- The fat triggers the small intestine to release chemicals to tell the brain that it's full.

- You should have loads of nonstarchy vegetables for antioxidants and satiety.

- A small amount of a low-glycemic, high-fiber carbs, such as lentils or berries, slowly releases sugar to the brain for energy so you can continue to focus. That will keep your blood sugar stable and insulin low so you can use stored fat for fuel.

Food is information. We want to make sure that we're telling our bodies to burn fat, build muscle and keep our energy steady and our focus spot-on.

Let's take a closer look.

# CLEAN, LEAN PROTEINS

Protein provides amino acids, which are our bodies' building blocks for muscle, hormones and neurotransmitters (the brain chemicals that we need for mood and focus). Protein is also what we need for great hair, skin and nails. When we consume carbs, we release insulin—and protein triggers the release of the key hormone glucagon, which helps balance out the effects of insulin, preventing insulin resistance and facilitating weight loss. The amino acids found in protein are critical for detoxification because they help escort the toxins out of our bodies. And, as we just saw, protein improves satiety. It's hard to feel full if you haven't had some protein. Protein can also lower sugar cravings.

Here are the proteins I want you to focus on:

| |
|---|
| Grass-fed beef |
| Hormone-free, free-range chicken and turkey |
| Pasture-fed lamb and pork |
| Pea–rice protein |
| Wild cold-water fish |
| Wild game |

## The Ground Rules for Protein

- **Enjoy lean red meat 3 or 4 times per week,** focusing on game and lamb. Get the rest of your protein from chicken, turkey, fish and my Virgin Diet Shakes.

- **For all animal protein, you are what you eat—and you are what you eat, ate.** That means if you're eating a commercially grown animal, it has probably eaten corn, soy or both, which means that *you* are eating corn, soy or both. So stay away from commercially farmed animals and concentrate on grass-fed beef, pasture-fed lamb and pork, and free-range chicken and turkey.

- **Game is a great choice because it hasn't been commercialized.** No hormones, no feed, no corn, no soy. You can feel pretty safe eating bison, elk, ostrich, wild venison and similar meats.

- **Cold-water wild fish only, please.** You don't want to eat what farm-raised fish are eating. And eat fish only from the safe list; otherwise, you're taking in mercury and other heavy metals that can create leaky gut, provoke inflammation and otherwise toxify your system. All three of those effects put weight on you that is nearly impossible to take off, so focus on safe fish.

- **Acceptable vegetarian proteins include pea, rice and hemp.** For more information on how to follow this program as a vegetarian or vegan, see the box below.

## SEAFOOD: WHAT'S SAFE AND WHAT'S NOT

### Highest Mercury Levels (avoid eating)

| | | |
|---|---|---|
| Grouper | Marlin | Shark |
| Mackarel (king) | Orange roughy | Swordfish |

## High Mercury (avoid eating or limit to one-two 6-oz servings a month)

| | | |
|---|---|---|
| Bass (saltwater) | Lobster (American, Maine) | Tuna (canned, white albacore) |
| Bluefish | Mahi mahi | Tuna (fresh bluefin, ahi) |
| Halibut (Atlantic) | Sea trout | |

## Lower Mercury (eat no more than six 6-oz servings per month)

| | | |
|---|---|---|
| Cod | Monkfish | Tuna (canned, chunk light) |
| Crab (Dungeness, blue, snow) | Snapper | Tuna (fresh, Pacific albacore) |

## Lowest Mercury (enjoy two or three 6-oz servings per week)

| | | |
|---|---|---|
| Anchovies | Flounder | Scallops |
| Butterfish | Halibut (Alaskan) | Shrimp |
| Calamari (squid) | Herring | Sole |
| Catfish | Lobster (spiny, rock) | Tilapia |
| Caviar (farmed) | Oysters | Trout (freshwater) |
| Clams | Pollock | Whitefish |
| Crab (king) | Salmon | |
| Crawfish/crayfish | Sardines | |

Data obtained from the websites of the U.S. Food and Drug Administration and the U.S. Environmental Protection Agency.

## If You Are Vegetarian or Vegan...

I'm going to be very straight with you: if I have a client eating a vegetarian or vegan diet for health reasons, I will encourage them to eat clean animal protein. Eating a vegetarian or vegan diet just is not as healthy as eating a more balanced, omnivorous diet. I know this from personal experience because I was a vegetarian for several years during my 20s. In that time, I had 10 percent higher body fat than I do now, despite the fact that I am 20 years older and work out about half as much now. Back then I also had cystic acne and low energy. So you do the math.

Of course, I completely respect if someone is vegetarian or vegan for spiritual reasons. So first, let me explain why I think animal protein is part of a healthy diet, and then I'll give you some nutritional support if you decide to continue with your vegetarian or vegan diet.

As I pointed out earlier, protein has major benefits for your metabolism: it improves satiety, slows down stomach emptying and suppresses ghrelin, the hormone produced by your stomach to trigger hunger. Protein is also critical for great hair, skin and nails; maintaining hormones; and building muscles. Now, when I recommend animal protein, I'm talking about clean, lean animal protein. I can understand your health concerns about eating meat from a corn-fed cow that's been stuck in a slaughterhouse covered in feces. I don't recommend eating that meat either. But nutritionally speaking, you would do well to have 1 or 2 servings per week of meat from a grass-fed cow that's been treated well, killed humanely and not choked with antibiotics and hormones. Other clean, lean proteins include wild salmon—not farm-raised fish!—other wild fish and free-range chicken. These are all healthy choices, and they're a critical part of an optimal diet.

When you're a vegetarian, you're failing to get the same quality of protein, and you're probably not getting the complete spectrum of all the amino acids you need. Remember, we digest or break down protein into amino acids, the building blocks of our body. So on a vegetarian diet, you *have* to supplement, and although I'm a big believer in supplements generally, I'm suspicious of any diet that requires supplements just to get the basics.

Now let's talk reactivity. Lacto-ovo vegetarians tend to eat a lot of dairy and eggs. What I see with most vegans is that they're eating a lot of soy and gluten. Both groups are getting the same two to four reactive foods multiple times a day. If this is your diet, the likelihood that you will have food reactions is very high. Because you're eating so many high-FI foods, you tend to have a higher risk for leaky gut. In addition, I see that many vegans have suppressed thyroid function because of their overconsumption of soy. Remember, thyroid is a key hormone for metabolism and weight loss.

Vegetarians and vegans are also eating lots of grains and legumes, foods that are high in lectins. We've already seen that lectins can challenge your immune system, interfere with your absorption of nutrients and perhaps create leptin resistance, which interferes with your hunger and full signals.

Another danger of eating a typical vegetarian diet that is rich in grains and legumes is phytates (or phytic acid), which *chelates,* or binds, with many key minerals, including calcium, iron, magnesium and zinc, making them virtually impossible for your body to absorb. Soy is especially rich in phytic acid, but you can find large amounts in corn, peanuts, whole wheat and rye as well.

Finally, a vegetarian/vegan diet is a high-carb diet. That can result in higher blood sugar and therefore higher insulin. Excess insulin can lead to insulin resistance, which in turn makes it hard to burn off fat and easy to store it, among other bad things that we will go into throughout the book.

So in a vegetarian/vegan diet, you're already eating foods that will be lower in certain nutrients or perhaps devoid of them altogether. Plus, a mainstay of your diet is *antinutrients.* You are eating more reactive foods that might aggravate leaky gut. You might also be deficient in vitamin B12, calcium, iron, zinc, riboflavin, thiamin and DHA. DHA is an essential omega-3 fatty acid that is critical for brain health. The highest source of DHA is from fish, although you can also get it from algae. Otherwise, your body will have to make it from nuts and seeds, especially flaxseed meal and hemp, but you have to eat a *lot* of nuts and seeds to produce as much DHA as you need.

Another problem is iron. Animal products are the best source of this essential mineral. You can get iron from a vegetarian diet, but it's not absorbed as well. On a vegetarian diet, it's hard to get enough zinc and vitamin B12 also. So here's another place that you have to supplement.

If you're avoiding all meat, poultry and fish, make sure you're supplementing with a good vegetarian multivitamin mineral formula that contains iron, zinc, calcium, magnesium and all the good B vitamins. Do a 25-hydroxy vitamin D test to evaluate your levels, and supplement with vitamin D3 to prevent a shortage. Vitamin D2 comes from plants, is not made by humans and is way less bioactive and stable than vitamin D3. Nearly all vitamin D3 comes from lanolin (i.e., sheep), but this is worth making the exception for, as vitamin D is a prohormone that is essential for strong bones and a healthy brain, heart and gastrointestinal tract. Also, be sure to take omega-3s from algae so you get enough DHA, and make sure you are taking extra vitamin B12. Check the Resources section on my website for recommendations on testing and supplements.

If you are a vegetarian or vegan, my Virgin Diet Shake, from pea–rice protein, is going to be a great protein-rich meal option for you. Make sure to eat a good blend of nuts, seeds, grains and legumes, especially lentils, which are the highest in protein. Quinoa is my favorite "grain" because it is not a true grain (it is more closely related to spinach and beets), it is gluten-free and it is higher in protein than other grains. But you can also have buckwheat, millet, rice, amaranth, arrowroot, sorghum and tapioca. Finally, whenever possible, consume soaked, sprouted or fermented foods to reduce the antinutrient impact of phytates and lectins.

# HEALTHY FATS

Fats have been falsely accused of being unhealthy for years, so I want to set the record straight. You need to eat fat to be healthy; in fact, you can't live without it. Fat reduces inflammation, keeps blood thinned and flowing well through your arteries and veins, supports membrane fluidity and keeps your hair glossy and your skin glowing. Ironically, you need to eat fat to burn fat. Plus, fat helps keep your hunger at bay and your mood balanced. Of course, to get these healthy benefits, you need to eat the right fats and cut out the wrong ones. You also need a good balance between the different types of mono- and polyunsaturated fats.

**You need to eat fat to burn fat.**

That's why one of my mantras for my clients is "make an oil change." Figuring out the fats might sound complicated, but if you follow the Virgin Diet, I have done the thinking (and balancing) for you.

Here are the healthy fats to focus on:

- Avocado
- Coconut milk or oil
- Olive oil, olives
- Palm fruit oil
- Raw nuts (no peanuts) and nut butter
- Raw seeds: chia, hemp, freshly ground flaxseed meal
- Sesame oil
- Wild cold-water fish

## Two Oil Rock Stars: Red Palm Fruit Oil and Coconut Oil

I want to give you a special shout-out for something that you probably haven't heard about before reading this book, even though it's common in other parts of the world.

I am in love with palm fruit oil. Produced in Malaysia and Africa, palm fruit oil has the most beautiful red color, thanks to carotenoids, a wonderful antioxidant that's the precursor to vitamin A. This type of oil is 15 times richer in beta-carotene than carrots, and it's also high in tocotrienols, the powerhouse component of vitamin E. Palm fruit oil helps reduce your risk of stroke and dementia, and it generally boosts your brain health. It's also important for heart health and great skin.

> Coconut oil is rich in lauric acid and caprylic acid.

Another great choice is coconut oil, which is rich in lauric acid and caprylic acid. These powerhouse fatty acids have antifungal, antibacterial and antiviral effects. Plus, coconut is rich in MCTs, medium-chain triglycerides, which help your body burn fat. It's a very stable oil, so you can cook with it at very high heats without damaging it. Do you see why I consider it an amazing food?

## GO NUTS!

Nuts are a terrific source of monounsaturated fats, and they're high in fiber, which is a big plus, but they're also high in lectins, phytates and other enzyme inhibitors. Here's a recipe to make nuts an even healthier choice:

1. Soak nuts overnight in water with sea salt and then drain the water.

2. Toss the nuts in cinnamon (or pumpkin pie spice) and unsweetened vanilla extract, or make them spicy and salty with curry powder and a little sea salt.

3. Spread the nuts onto a cookie sheet.

4. Bake at 140 degrees for 8 hours.

5. Cool and then store in the fridge.

# HIGH-FIBER, LOW-GLYCEMIC CARBS

We actually can live without carbohydrates, but our mood and energy will suffer a bit for it. By eating what I call "slow low" carbs, you will keep a steady supply of energy going to your brain to help you stay focused and energetic. *Slow* is because they are higher in fiber, which means that their sugar is released more slowly. *Low* is because they are generally lower on the glycemic index. Finally, whenever possible, consume soaked, sprouted or fermented grains and beans to reduce the antinutrient impact of phytates and lectins. Fruit falls into this category, too, so remember to choose from low- and moderate-glycemic fruits. I will make it easy for you: toss berries into your shake, and if you need that afternoon snack, try an apple with almond or cashew nut butter. Here are more high-fiber, low-glycemic carbs to choose from:

| | | |
|---|---|---|
| Adzuki beans | Great Northern beans | Oat bran |
| Beets | Jicama | Okra |
| Black beans | Kidney beans | Pumpkin |
| Brown rice | Legumes | Quinoa |
| Brown rice pasta or quinoa pasta | Lentils | Split peas |
| Brown rice wraps | Lima beans | Squash (acorn, butternut, winter) |

| Carrots | Millet | Sweet potato or yam |
|---|---|---|
| Chick peas (garbanzos) | Mung beans | Tomatoes |
| Cowpeas | Navy beans | Turnip |
| French beans | | White beans |

## THE CASE FOR CARROTS

Carrots really straddle both the nonstarchy and the starchy groups. They are higher on the glycemic index than most vegetables (meaning that they have some natural sugar that quickly drives your blood sugar up), but they aren't a full-blown starch because they have only 13 grams of carbs per cup (most starchy carbs have 2 to 4 times that much). After all, carrots have only 6 grams of sugar (again, most carbs score higher), plus they are rich in fiber, potassium, vitamin C and beta-carotene, all of which we love.

What's my verdict? Carrots are great to have as part of your crudités or grated onto a salad—that is, eat them raw and along with other foods. What you don't want to do is juice them, cook them, bake them as a cake or snack on just carrots. (Remember the fat-free craze when everyone was snacking on baby carrots all day long? What a sneaky way to get sugar and starch!)

## Grappling with Grains

Do we need grains in our diet? Despite what you may have heard else-where, the answer is no. All grains have lectins, a type of protein that can challenge your immune system, interfere with your absorption of nutrients and perhaps cause resistance to the hormone leptin, which regulates feelings of hunger and fullness. Leptin resistance means you can't tell when you're full, so you keep on eating even when you've had enough.

**We can exist perfectly fine on vegetables, fruits, nuts and seeds and clean protein.**

On the plus side, grains are a great source of fiber, especially when you choose less refined ver-sions, such as steel-cut oats rather than instant oatmeal, or quinoa as opposed to white rice. So eating the grains that I've recommended for the Virgin Diet can be a healthy and delicious choice.

Legumes have lectins, too, but there are so many benefits to legumes that I allow them in moderate amounts. Legumes are rich in fiber and very low on the glycemic index—unlike grains, which, although high in fiber, are also higher on the glycemic index. Grains are also relatively new to our food supply—

**Too much healthy food is unhealthy!**

we only started eating them 5,000 to 10,000 years ago—and we can exist perfectly fine (and, I believe, better) on vegetables, fruits, nuts and seeds and clean animal and fish protein.

That said, you are allowed sweet potatoes and some root veggies, some legumes and even some grains in limited amounts. But don't go over-board: too much healthy food is unhealthy! Grains, legumes and starchy veggies can be incorporated into a healthy diet if they are not eaten in excess, which means 1 to 4 servings per day (1 serving is approximately half a cup).

## SOAKING AND SPROUTING

There are two things that you can do to reduce the lectin and phytate content in grains and legumes: soak them or sprout them. These processes reduce the antinutrient loads and make grains and legumes somewhat healthier and much easier to digest. Soak your beans overnight in very warm water, approximately 140 degrees. If you are buying canned beans, those have already been soaked. You can purchase a sprouting unit to sprout your beans or grains (see the Resources section on my website).

## NONSTARCHY VEGETABLES

To get a variety of antioxidants, I want you to eat from the rainbow of nonstarchy vegetables. The antioxidants in vegetables help reduce

> Vegetables help reduce inflammation and lower oxidative stress.

inflammation and lower oxidative stress which can help slow down the aging process, and different antioxidants are associated with different colors. For example, you can load up on sulforaphane when you eat dark green broccoli, and you'll get a lot of vitamin C from bright red peppers. The broader the variety of veggies you consume, the more likely you'll get a good range of antioxidants. Nonstarchy veggies are also a great source of fiber and can help add bulk to your diet without many additional calories. Here are some of my favorites:

| | | |
|---|---|---|
| Arugula | Chicory | Mushrooms |
| Artichokes | Chives | Mustard greens |
| Asparagus | Collard greens | Onions |
| Bamboo shoots | Coriander | Parsley |
| Bean sprouts | Dandelion greens | Radicchio |
| Beet greens | Eggplant | Radishes |
| Bell peppers (red, yellow, green) | Endive | Shallots |
| Broccoli | Fennel | Spaghetti squash |
| Brussels sprouts | Garlic | Spinach |
| Cabbage | Green beans | Summer squash |
| Carrots (see The Case for Carrots) | Jalapeño peppers | Swiss chard |
| Cassava | Kale | Turnip greens |
| Cauliflower | Kohlrabi | Watercress |
| Celery | Lettuce | Zucchini |

## BEWARE OF THE NIGHTSHADES

You can eat most vegetables on a regular basis without worrying about food intolerance, but sometimes the nightshades can cause you trouble: eggplants, peppers, potatoes and tomatoes. The problem comes from their lectin content. (Lectins are a type of protein that can interfere with the absorption of nutrients.) Be a little cautious if you notice any reactions to nightshades, usually noticed as joint pain—yet another reason to keep a food journal.

## Figuring Out Your Fruit

The glycemic index is a gauge of how quickly your body converts a fruit, vegetable or grain into blood sugar. (See pages 128–129 for more on the glycemic index.) Sometimes it can be misleading, but I find it really useful when it comes to fruit. To maintain the healthy, steady levels of blood sugar that are optimal for your weight, I want you to focus on low- and moderate-glycemic fruits. As a general rule, avoid high-glycemic fruits, especially during Cycle 1, when you are seriously trying to retune your metabolism. The high-glycemic fruits are just loaded with sugar—you might as well have a candy bar. (No, I do *not* mean that it's okay to have a candy bar!)

### LOW-GLYCEMIC INDEX FRUITS (FAVOR THESE)

| | | |
|---|---|---|
| Blackberries | Elderberries | Loganberries |
| Blueberries | Gooseberries | Raspberries |
| Boysenberries | | Strawberries |

### MODERATE-GLYCEMIC INDEX FRUITS (EAT IN MODERATION)

| | | |
|---|---|---|
| Apples | Limes | Peaches |
| Apricots | Melons | Pear |
| Cherries | Nectarines | Persimmons |
| Grapefruit | Oranges | Plums |
| Kiwi | Passion fruit | Pomegranates |
| Lemons | | Tangerines |

### HIGH-GLYCEMIC INDEX FRUITS (AVOID)

| | | |
|---|---|---|
| Bananas | Mango | Pineapple |
| Grapes | Papaya | Watermelon |

# STEP 3: DRINK VIRGIN DIET SHAKES

I teach everyone to start the day with a smoothie. Why? I find that most
people eat dessert for breakfast: muffins, buttered toast, pancakes with

syrup, toaster pastries, etc.—these foods spike your blood sugar and are really desserts. A muffin is just a cupcake. Look at what it's wrapped in. Plus, almost every breakfast food contains gluten, eggs, dairy or soy. Breakfast sets the metabolic tone for the day. If you eat dessert for breakfast and get your blood sugar rolling, it will roll all day long. You'll start with a big, sugar-rush spike, and then by midmorning, you are going to crash. You're going to reach for more dessert, then away you go. You're off to the races, and it will be a bad race.

Now, just because you're not pigging out on starches and dairy doesn't mean you don't need a substantial breakfast. Eating the right combination of foods in the morning means that you will lose more weight and keep it off.

## THREE WEEKS TO THINNER AND YOUNGER

### Week 1: Jump Start Week

- 2 shakes, 1 meal, optional snack

### Weeks 2 and 3: Healing Weeks

- 1 shake, 2 meals, optional snack
(You can do 2 shakes if you prefer.)

I recently read a study that showed that people who ate 600 calories for breakfast lost more weight and kept it off than the skimpy breakfast eaters who stuck to 200 calories. So, I like people to eat a substantial, balanced breakfast, generally around 400 to 500 calories. People tell me silly things like they're not hungry for breakfast, or they don't have time for breakfast. I tell them, "If you don't have time, make time." One of the most common habits I see with my clients who are struggling with weight loss is the bad habit of skipping breakfast. By the way, once you start eating breakfast every morning, you will start to get hungry for it.

This is a good thing: you want your metabolism fired up in the morning. Remember that my Virgin Diet Plate includes clean, lean protein at each meal, including breakfast, for a reason. A recent study compared the metabolic impact of a high-carb breakfast with a high-protein breakfast and found that a higher protein breakfast slowed down stomach emptying and kept ghrelin suppressed, which improved satiety.[26] If you are satiated, you will not feel the need to reach for those darn 100-calorie snack packs every few hours!

> Eating the right combination of foods in the morning means that you will lose more weight and keep it off.

The easiest way to solve this problem is to start the day with a smoothie. Studies are clear on the benefits. To cite just one example, a 2003 study in the *International Journal of Obesity and Related Metabolic Disorders* found that by using meal-replacement shakes, "these types of interventions can safely and effectively produce significant sustainable weight loss and improve weight-related risk factors of disease."[27]

> You want your metabolism fired up in the morning.

Make a Virgin Diet Shake. Then I know you are getting everything you need. Virgin Diet Shakes contain a blend of protein (to boost metabolism and satiety), fiber (to cleanse and support your GI tract and fight hunger), healthy fats (to reduce inflammation and improve satiety) and berries (super antioxidants to prevent aging and help your system heal). I've included my basic recipe plus two variations here. If you like, throw in a tablespoon of nut butter. You can also add in some kale or spinach (fresh or frozen). I think you're a rock star if you add the green stuff, and you won't even taste it (especially the spinach). And you'll be boosting your nutrients and giving yourself a great start for the day. Since scoop sizes vary by protein powder brand and manufacturer, aim for 20 to 25 grams of protein per shake.

## THE VIRGIN DIET SHAKE

SERVES

1–2 scoops vegan pea–rice protein powder* (See the Resources section on my website.)

1–2 tablespoons** fiber (fiber blend, chia seeds, hemp seeds, freshly ground flaxseed meal or nut butter)

½–1 cup organic frozen berries

1 cup liquid (water, unsweetened coconut milk*** or coconut water)

| I LIKE MY SHAKE THINNER! | I LIKE MY SHAKE THICKER! |
|---|---|
| 1–2 scoops protein | 1–2 scoops protein |
| 1 serving fiber | 1 serving fiber |
| ½ cup organic frozen fruit | 1 serving chia seeds, hemp seeds or freshly ground flaxseeds |
| 10 ounces liquid | 1 cup organic frozen fruit |
| 1 cup spinach | 8 ounces liquid |
| | Ice cubes |

* Aim for 20-25 grams of protein per shake.

** I really want you to pump up your fiber, so build up to those 2 tablespoons per shake.

*** I recommend So Delicious unsweetened coconut milk. If you use canned coconut milk, choose the light version and dilute ¼ cup coconut milk with ¾ cup water.

## "HELP! I CAN'T DO THE SHAKES!"

I am a big proponent of using high-quality meal-replacement shakes to replace 1 or 2 meals per day. The research is clear that people who do this lose more weight *and* keep it off. I like shakes because they make it easy to get in a great balanced breakfast, and I find that this is the meal that most people struggle with, either because they just aren't hungry, they don't have "time" (make time, please!), or they are used to eating dessert for breakfast. A shake solves all of these problems and removes the opportunities for bad decisions that can also take you down. For all of these reasons, the Virgin Diet Shake is a critical part of the program.

But if you just can't do a shake, then you can have lunch or dinner for breakfast. Yep, that's right. It may seem strange the first day or two, and then it will be your new normal.

## WHAT TO LOOK FOR IN YOUR SHAKE

- No artificial sweeteners
- 5 grams or less of sugar
- No whey, dairy, milk solids, egg or soy (Soy lecithin is okay.)
- No maltodextrin
- 5 grams or more of fiber
- pea, rice and/or potato and chlorella protein (See the Resources section on my website.)
- Sugar alcohols (Stevia is acceptable.)

# STEP 4: FOLLOW THE GOLDEN RULES OF MEAL TIMING

An important part of the Virgin Diet isn't just what you eat, it's when you eat. When you eat, you raise blood sugar. When you raise blood sugar, you raise insulin. When you raise insulin, you shut down fat burning. Yes, when we are digesting, we are boosting metabolism. But we're not boosting metabolism enough to compensate for the calories that we're eating.

> **It's important to eat only every 4 to 6 hours.**

That's why it's important to eat only every 4 to 6 hours. Because you're getting clean, lean protein; healthy fats; a little bit of high-fiber, low-glycemic carbs; and loads of nonstarchy vegetables in every meal on this plan, you'll have a nice steady release of blood sugar to your brain. Your insulin levels stay down so you can access stored fat for fuel. You feel great. You feel energized.

If you must, have 2 meals, an afternoon snack and then a final meal, but if you can, get yourself down to 3 meals. Ultimately, you'll feel better, look better and lose weight faster. So if you wake up at 6, you should eat breakfast by 7, have lunch between 11 and 1 and eat dinner between 5 and 7. If you are eating the earlier lunch at 11 and a later dinner at 7 or after, then you can do that afternoon snack at 3.

There are two exceptions to this rule. First, if you are an athlete and actively increasing your muscle mass, then you will eat every 4 hours and have 4 meals each day, rather than 3. This is how I helped Brandon Routh pack on 20 pounds of muscle when he starred as Superman. The other exception is if you have to eat every 2 to 3 hours because of reactive hypoglycemia or a known medical condition. If you have to do this, that's okay, although I have found that I can spread most people to

3 hours and then 4 hours so they end up eating 2 meals, a snack and then another meal on this program.

## FOLLOW THE GOLDEN RULES

- Drink your Virgin Diet Shake within an hour of waking up. If you're working out first thing, you can have half your shake before and half after.

- Eat every 4 to 6 hours.

- Stop eating 2 to 3 hours before bed. Note: That does *not* mean you get to go to bed later!

## DOING WATER RIGHT

- When you get up: 16 ounces

- 30 to 60 minutes before each meal: 16 ounces

- During a meal: limit to 4 to 8 ounces. Start drinking water again 60 minutes after each meal.

- Before bed: 8 ounces

- Daily total: 64 ounces minimum; more if you are in a hot climate, exercise heavily or are heavier. You should be drinking approximately half your weight in ounces.

Keep a water bottle with you to continue to drink between meals so you drink enough. Thirty minutes before each meal, start limiting fluids to no more than 8 ounces of water until an hour after the meal. That's because having fluids with your food

> diletes your stomach acid. That bedtime water is really helpful, too, to prevent nighttime cravings. According to a study done at the University of Washington, drinking 8 ounces of water at bedtime can shut down your evening hunger pangs.[28]

# STEP 5: STAY HYDRATED

Water is queen for weight loss. Water will help you get healthy and lose weight faster than any other single substance. Do you know how often you're not hungry, but you're really thirsty?

For some reason, nature endowed us with a terrible thirst monitor. By the time you know you're thirsty, it's too late—you're already dehydrated. I have no idea why our bodies evolved this way—maybe to survive in water-scarce climates—but it's crucial to stay ahead of the curve by hydrating *before* you feel thirsty.

This isn't just a health issue, it's also a weight-loss issue. Even mild dehydration of 1 to 2 percent can raise cortisol levels. Cortisol is a stress hormone,

**Water is queen for weight loss.**

and one of the things it can do is cause you to store more fat around your waist. So dehydration can block fat burning, undoing all the good you're doing by eating right and exercising. We need water to burn fat.

Did you know that our bodies should be 70 percent water? Most people are down at 45 to 50 percent. Dehydration is yet another risk factor for inflammation. Drinking water throughout the day is the solution.

Now, a lot of people think that any kind of fluid is the same as water. It's not. Coffee, tea and soft drinks are highly acidic and actually dehydrate you. You need to drink even more water to overcome the dehy-drating effects of the coffee or tea.

Not all water is created equal. If it started out as pure spring water but you're drinking it out of plastic bottles, now it's pure spring water plus phthalates (a toxic ingredient in the plastic that may disrupt hormones and promote obesity). Not to mention the landfill issue and the fact that you're creating a huge carbon footprint each time you drink one. So no more plastic bottles.

Get creative to inspire yourself to drink more water. Try sparkling water (get the kind in the glass bottles) with a little lime. Or make what I call "spa water." I loved going to the spa and getting those special waters with cucumbers, oranges, lemon, lime and maybe a little mint or basil. One day I realized that I could get that spa experience at home—and you can, too. Use whatever essence you love.

Here's the rest of my guide to healthy water intake:

- Put a water filter on every tap in your house.
- Track your water intake in your food journal.
- Water will curb your appetite anyway, but if you want some more help, throw 5 to 10 grams of fiber into some water and drink it 30 minutes before your meals. (See the Resources section on my website.)

## STEP 6: LOAD UP ON LOW-FI AND HEALING FOODS

Food is here to nourish us. It's here to rebuild us. And it's here to heal. Along with pulling out the high-FI foods that create adverse reactions, we'll bring in foods that heal.

## LOW-FI FOODS

First, here are the key low-FI foods. I want you to eat these on a regular basis. These low-FI foods are the least reactive foods I know, and they will help your body heal:

> Food is here to nourish us. It's here to rebuild us. And it's here to heal.

### PROTEINS

Hormone-free, free-range chicken and turkey

Pasture-fed lamb

Pea, rice and/or hemp protein

Wild cold-water fish

### NONSTARCHY VEGETABLES

**They all fit in here, but especially focus in on:**

| | |
|---|---|
| Broccoli | Deep green leafy vegetables |
| Cabbage | Kale |
| Cauliflower | Spinach |

### FRUIT

| | |
|---|---|
| Apples | Blueberries |

## FATS

| | |
|---|---|
| Avocado | Extra-virgin olive oil |
| Chia seeds | Freshly ground flaxseed meal |
| Coconut oil and coconut milk | Palm fruit oil |

## HIGH-FIBER STARCHY CARBS

| | |
|---|---|
| Brown rice | Quinoa |
| Lentils | Sweet potatoes |

## FERMENTED FOODS

These have been used a lot in ancient times and in many of the Middle Eastern and Asian cultures. Sadly, the ones we know, like sauerkraut, aren't necessarily so healing anymore because they aren't prepared in the traditional way. But when you ferment a food—or soak it or sprout it—it vastly reduces the lectins and phytates, and it may even eliminate them altogether.

Fermentation is a little bit like predigesting your food. Hard-to-digest elements, such as lactose, are consumed in the fermentation process, making everything easier to digest and lowering the overall sugar content. Fermented foods also contain beneficial bacteria that act as pre- and probiotics. That helps feed the healthy bacteria in your gut. That is your warrior defense system.

Many fermented foods in more traditional cultures don't ever make it into our consciousness. You've probably never been offered fermented camel's milk, but they drink it in the Middle East all the time. Rakfisk is salted fermented trout from Scandinavia, and it's also very healthy.

Dark chocolate is generally fermented. Isn't that great to hear? Pickled ginger—the kind you get in a Japanese restaurant—is also fermented. So is kimchi, the Korean cabbage dish, and traditionally prepared sauerkraut. Fermented fish sauces can be great, but be careful: they often contain gluten. Kombucha, the green tea, is fermented, but make sure there's no sugar added.

Yogurt is fermented, so in Cycle 3, if you can handle some dairy, you can have some Greek-style yogurt and kefir. In Cycle 1, you can even get a starter kit and make coconut-milk kefir, a phenomenal prebiotic and probiotic fizzy cocktail that is good for your gut (see the Resources section on my website for more information).

Now, when I say *fermented*, I mean soaking, fermenting, sprouting and pickling—the whole traditional process. You want to avoid commercially fermented foods because usually they are just preserved in vinegar after being run through a lactobacterial salt slurry.

## HEALING FOODS

Healing foods soothe and heal the gastrointestinal tract, reduce inflammation, balance blood sugar, support healthy gut bacteria and help you have poops that you can be proud of 2 or 3 times per day. Some of the most powerful healing foods are vegetables. There are so many amazing, different kinds that you can add into your diet.

> Some of the most powerful healing foods are vegetables.

Look for color in your fruits and vegetables—that way you're sure to get a variety of healing vitamins and minerals. The exception to that would be cauliflower. Along with cabbage and broccoli, cauliflower is a sulforaphane rock star. (For more on the benefits of sulforaphane, see the entries for cabbage and broccoli below.)

Here's a long list of healing foods and spices. Use them to vary your diet and heal your body at the same time.

**Apples:** Apples contain pectin, which helps heal your gut. They're also rich in fiber.

**Artichokes:** Loaded with antioxidants and fiber and rich in the super antioxidant glutathione, this thistle also supports healthy liver function. Because your liver metabolizes fat, you want it in peak condition to facilitate weight loss.

**Avocado:** Whether sliced into a salad or mashed up with lime, cilantro and salsa, avocado supports immune function and libido. It's also a very healthy source of monounsaturated fats.

**Beets:** This food is rich in betacyanin, which helps lower homocysteine, an amino acid that increases your risk of heart disease and stroke. Beets also help cleanse your blood and are great for liver health.

**Blueberries/berries:** These nutrient-dense fruits are high in fiber and antioxidants, which help heal your digestive tract, keep it functioning in peak condition and help reverse the aging process.

**Broccoli:** One of my favorite healing foods, broccoli is high in sulforaphane and rich in antioxidants, which help prevent cancer and is a powerful weapon in the antiaging battle. Broccoli is also high in fiber, which will help you eliminate food and keep your digestive tract functioning in top condition. Broccoli is a true superfood: eat it on a regular basis.

**Cabbage:** Whether eaten raw as slaw or boiled up in fragrant soup, cabbage kills Helicobacter pylori, the bacteria that causes peptic ulcers. Cabbage is also rich in sulfur, which supports Cycle 2 detoxification.

**Chia seeds:** These are high in fiber and rich in omega-3s. If you like thicker protein shakes, chia seeds are a great addition.

**Cilantro:** This green, leafy plant helps chelate heavy metals; that is, it pulls killer metals, such as lead and mercury from your blood and helps your body flush them out. Without that toxic burden, your immune system heals, and your food intolerance evaporates.

**Cinnamon:** This delicious spice is great for balancing blood sugar.

**Coconut:** An antiviral food, coconut contains medium-chain triglycerides (MCTs), which are good for metabolism and circulation. It's also thermogenic, which means it stimulates metabolism to promote weight loss. Coconut also helps reduce microbial overgrowth, fungus and intestinal yeast, and it's a high-antioxidant food.

**Curcumin:** This is a major anti-inflammatory supplement as well as a terrific antioxidant and blood sugar balancer. You can take it as a supplement or find it in turmeric, so spice up those curries or sprinkle some on chicken, veggies or quinoa.

**Dandelion greens:** Throw some yummy dandelion greens into your salad because they have plenty of the soluble fiber called inulin, which is a great prebiotic; they help feed the probiotic bacteria in your intestines; and they stimulate bile production, which will help you better emulsify your fats and stay regular. It is also a natural anti-inflammatory.

**Extra-virgin olive oil:** This heart-healthy oil supports healthy blood pressure and cholesterol levels. (I like to think they named it after me, but maybe I'm kidding myself?)

**Flaxseed meal:** This gut-healing food is both anti-inflammatory and high in fiber. It has lignans, which are great for modulating hormone response. It's also rich in omega-3 fats.

**Garlic:** This pungent herb is a powerful blood thinner, antimicrobial, antifungal and antiviral. It thins and detoxifies your blood while fighting bacteria and fungus. Garlic is great for zapping the bad bacteria while supporting the good, so it helps reduce microbial overgrowth, fungus and intestinal yeast.

**Ginger:** Gut-healing, anti-inflammatory and anti-ulcer, ginger is also good for aiding digestion. A delicious substitute for tamari when you're making fish, it will pleasantly stimulate your taste buds with its spicy flavor. That taste explosion makes spicy foods more filling than bland ones, so if you're feeling hungry, try a cup of ginger tea.

**Green tea:** Drinking green tea supports healthy gut bacteria and boosts metabolism. This wonder beverage contains theanine, which raises GABA, a calming brain chemical that combats depression, promotes good sleep and helps your body overcome food intolerance.

**Lentils:** High in fiber and protein, these are one of my favorite carbs because instead of causing your blood sugar to spike and crash, they release their sugars very slowly. In other words, eat some lentils, and you'll feel satiated and energetic for a long time after your meal.

**Oregano:** This Italian spice helps reduce microbial overgrowth, fungus and yeast. Plus, it's high in antioxidants, which will help you reduce your inflammatory load.

**Palm fruit oil:** If you need to cook something at high heat, this is the oil to use because even extreme temperatures cannot destroy its beneficial qualities. As we have seen, palm fruit oil contains the perfect balance of saturated and polyunsaturated fats and is rich in carotenoids and tocotrienols, more antiaging chemicals.

**Pomegranate:** A great source of ellagic acid, pomegranates are also a terrific way to consume polyphenols, a powerful antioxidant that fights aging and cancer.

**Red onions:** Another natural antihistamine, these are also rich in quercetin, a flavonoid that supports your immune system while fighting cancer and heart disease.

**Red peppers:** These colorful veggies are rich in vitamin C and are a natural antihistamine. Fighting histamines helps you combat inflammation. Red peppers are also terrific for supporting your adrenal glands. Out-of-balance adrenals might overproduce cortisol, a stress hormone that causes you to store fat.

**Rosemary:** Rosemary fights inflammation and is a major antioxidant.

**Sauerkraut:** One of the few fermented foods that has no gluten, dairy or yeast, sauerkraut supports healthy gut bacteria.

**Sea salt:** Use it sparingly, but do use some because it's rich in minerals. However, avoid regular table salt like the plague because it will only set you up for high blood pressure, heart disease and kidney problems.

**Seafood, especially salmon, sardines, sole and scallops:** These foods are gut healing and full of omega-3s, the healing fats that combat inflammation and support your metabolism.

**Sweet potato:** Rich in carotenoids (antioxidants, anticancer) and fiber, this vegetable is a natural way to satisfy your sweet tooth. It's moderate on the glycemic index, which means it won't make your blood sugar spike and crash but will help you feel satisfied and full for a while.

**Xylitol:** The only therapeutic sweetener in existence, this natural sugar alcohol helps with your acid–alkaline balance (which is good for weight loss) while supporting your bone mineralization (anti-osteoporosis). Unlike other sugars, it doesn't feed yeast (see Chapter 3) and helps prevent dental caries.

## STEP 7: EAT PLENTY OF FABULOUS FIBER

Fiber is my favorite health secret. The average American eats 5 to 14 grams of fiber per day, which is not nearly enough. You should have 50 grams of fiber per day. However, I don't want to take you from 5 to 50 overnight. We want to slowly increase your fiber so your body can adjust to it. Every other day, add another 5 grams of fiber from food or a fiber supplement blend until you're at 50. As you do so, you *must* follow my water schedule. I can't tell you how miserable you're going to feel if you don't. If at any point along the path of increasing your intake you feel "stuck," hold off on increasing your fiber intake until that passes (and I mean that literally).

Why do I love fiber so much? Fiber is the ultimate weight-loss tool. It slows down stomach emptying, which suppresses ghrelin, the hormone that sends hunger signals from your stomach to your brain. Fiber also helps stabilize your blood sugar levels, which lowers your insulin levels so you can use stored fat for fuel.

> **Fiber is the ultimate weight-loss tool.**

There are two kinds of fiber: soluble and insoluble. Most high-fiber foods contain a mix of both types. Soluble fiber is found in apples, berries and flaxseed meal. Insoluble fiber is mainly found in whole grains and vegetables.

Soluble fiber is great because it is very soothing to the gut and helps heal it. Soluble fiber particles are like little sponges. They attract water and form a jelly sponge. You want things to go slow in the stomach, and fiber also helps slow things down. It can also raise HDL (the good cholesterol) even while it lowers LDL (the bad cholesterol) by interfering with its absorption. How incredible is that?

Once food hits the intestines, though, especially the large intestine, you don't want food hanging out. If you made a bowel movement in the toilet, would you leave it sitting there? No, it would stink. You don't want it sitting in your intestines either. Here's where insoluble fiber is very useful. Once soluble fiber has given bulk to the stool, insoluble fiber has a laxative effect that speeds up the passage of food and waste through your gut.

Fiber is also detoxifying, and it feeds good gut bacteria. I'm telling you, if this were a drug, everyone would be taking it. This is one of those secrets that only nutritionists tend to know. Let's not keep it a secret anymore.

## SLEEP WELL, DESTRESS…AND LOSE WEIGHT!

Getting a good night's sleep and letting go of stress are actually crucial to weight loss. I go into more detail about how to add some stress busters to your life when we get to Cycle 3, but if you're eager to get started on that part of the Virgin Diet now, check out the helpful tools I recommend for stress and sleep in the Resources section at www.thevirgindiet.com/resources.

## MAKING IT THROUGH THE FIRST FEW DAYS

My favorite way to run a weight-loss program is with a forum. During the first 3 to 4 days, people absolutely whine and cry. They miss their food. They really crave their problem foods. And that may well happen to you.

But remember, those foods are holding your health hostage. I always tell clients in the forum, "That's fantastic," when I hear about their cravings—because that means that these were reactive foods for them, and cravings mean that the program is working. So, in those first few days, I want you to reframe your experience. When you feel like you're dying for a sweet dessert or might kill for some macaroni and cheese, imagine that I'm telling you (or tell yourself), "That's fantastic." Those

**Your body is telling you that you have a serious problem.**

feelings should tell you all you need to know. Your body is telling you that you have a serious problem, and it's up to you to pay attention.

> **By the end of the first week, the cravings will be gone, and so will the bloat.**

I've had people tell me, "I gave up the soy and the gluten, but I couldn't give up my cheese."

I say, "Honey, that's the one you have to give up. You have to stop the cheese."

I think that's what you'll see, too. Those foods that you just can't go without are the ones that are causing all of your problems. They are your weight-loss culprits. They are the reason your IgG antibodies are just crying out for you to eat some more so your immune system can zap them—and then start the inflammatory process all over again. Remember, it's only 21 days!

So, yes. The first couple of days you will think, *Oh my gosh. It's killing me to go without my cheese (or soy or whatever).* That's great. Each day will get easier. You will get past that third, fourth or fifth day, and then you will never want to go back. I see it all the time. When people get to the end of the first week, they are so thrilled. They are so happy. They are so excited.

If you make it through the "tearing out your hair" phase, by the end of the first week, the cravings will be gone, and so will the bloat. Your energy levels will be amazing. You will say, "Wow," and you will keep on saying it until 21 days have passed and you are 10 pounds lighter and look 10 years younger. Keep your eye on *that* prize and prevail.

 ## YES, A LITTLE BIT MATTERS

Now, here's how we know that this diet plan is about nutrition and chemistry and not about calories. You might easily be tempted to steal a bite of someone's dessert, use a spoonful of Caesar dressing or order the soy-marinated duck at your favorite restaurant. In terms of calories, these tiny amounts of forbidden foods might seem negligible, and on a traditional diet based on the archaic bank account model of "calories in, calories out," that might be true.

However, that's why traditional diets don't work. If you've got weight that won't come off, it's almost certainly because your system is out of whack, and if that is the case, even tiny amounts of dairy, egg, gluten or soy can keep the weight on and hold your symptoms in place. You wouldn't give a heroin addict just a tiny bit of the drug, would you?

**Traditional diets don't work.**

You would understand that in order to heal, the person's body has to become completely free of the problem substance.

You're in the same position. If you want your body to heal, you can't be 99 percent free of the top 7 high-FI foods. You have to achieve 100 percent for 21 days. That's not me talking, it's biology. I don't make the rules—I just enforce them!

## WHAT TO DO IF A LITTLE HIGH-FI SNEAKS IN . . .

Now, this is *not* a license to sneak in tiny bits of forbidden food. Even the smallest bite of baked goods or the tiniest spoonful of dairy can sabotage all your good, healing efforts.

However, if you make a mistake and don't discover it until later, you might not have to start the Virgin Diet all over again. In Cycle 2, when you challenge the potentially healthy 4 high-FI foods, just make sure you wait 21 days before you challenge the food you inadvertently ate. For instance, if you ate soy on

day 7 by accident, wait until at least day 28 before testing soy.
You want 21 free days before testing any particular food.

This is why it is critical to keep that food journal that I insist
you keep (and I mean insist—this is not optional!). If you notice
that last night's dinner didn't make you feel stellar, you can do
some research to figure out why.

# THE FIVE FUNDAMENTALS FOR FAST AND LASTING FAT LOSS

For the better part of 3 decades, I've been working with people trying
to lose weight. And here is what I've learned about how to help people
lose weight and keep it off:

1. **Lose fat fast.** We've got this covered in Cycle 1. If you pull all
   7 high-FI foods from your diet, you will lose up to 7 pounds
   in 7 days. That's the fastest you can lose weight and still be healthy.

2. **Weigh and measure yourself each week and write down
   whatever you want to track.** What you measure, you can
   improve. Each week, note your weight; the measurements of
   your waist, hips and thighs; and whatever else you want to
   track or improve: your water intake, your supplement schedule,
   your bowel movements (seriously!). (You can find a tracking
   guide and journal pages at www.thevirgindiet.com/journal and
   www.thevirgindiet.com/weighttracker.

3. **Get support and be accountable.** There have been a ton of studies showing that support is crucial for weight loss, and my 2-plus decades in the business confirm that. I think support is so important that I've set up an online support forum on my website. Go to www.thevirgindiet.com/forum right now and check it out. Support forces you to be accountable, which is key. It's too easy to slip when you're the only one who knows what you have and haven't done. Find a coach, friend, group or accountability buddy.

4. **Rechallenge and customize.** That's what Cycle 2 is for. You'll figure out exactly which foods you can tolerate and which ones are likely to start up the symptoms and put on the pounds. You can keep rechallenging and customizing every 3 months if you like because foods that you cannot tolerate now may work for you once your system has further healed.

5. **Plan for maintenance.** Maintenance is what Cycle 3 is all about. Once you've hit your ideal weight, you need to keep planning how to maintain it. Make it personal. If you hate going to the gym, buy some home equipment. If there's no refrigerator at work for your healthy lunch choices, buy a thermos, bring in a cooler, locate a restaurant you can order from or choose some lunch items that don't need to be refrigerated. You get the idea. Figure out what you need to do to maintain the great results you've created for yourself on the Virgin Diet.

THREE CYCLES TO LOSE WEIGHT FOR GOOD

# HOW THE VIRGIN DIET WORKED FOR ME

Kelly Taylor
Age 34

McBain,
Michigan

**Height:**
5'10"

**Starting Weight:**
185 pounds

**Waist:** 40"
**Hips:** 45.25"

**Current Weight:**
172.2 pounds

**Waist:** 37.5"
**Hips:** 42.5"

**Lost:** 12.8 pounds

I'm a wife and mom of three. While I've been on the Virgin Diet, I've been working full-time. I've got a lot on my plate, but I'm so glad that I did the Virgin Diet!

I think the biggest physical change is just more energy. I also feel more mentally alert and have the energy to both physically and mentally engage my husband and kids in the evenings after work. I definitely feel more confident, and my clothes fit better.

My biggest takeaway is that vegetables and salads are okay to eat and even good tasting. I've never been a huge veggie fan—green beans and carrots being the extent before, for the most part—but they are growing on me.

The Virgin Diet Shakes and the Virgin Diet Plate, I think, were huge factors in my success with the program. Before I didn't usually even eat breakfast, so the Virgin Diet Shake for breakfast has been great. I really like that the exercise isn't overwhelming, too. Fifteen minutes and done—even with a busy schedule, I can usually fit that in.

Thanks for such a great program!

I'm so excited for you! You've just finished Cycle 1 of the Virgin Diet, which means that you've dropped weight and look years younger! I'm betting that you have more energy, great skin and healthy hair and that you have discovered how great life can be when you drop the high-FI foods that have been disrupting your digestion and sapping your health.

Cycle 1 was all about taking foods out. We pulled the top 7 high-FI foods and gave your system a chance to heal. Cycle 2 is about putting foods in—slowly so we can truly figure out what foods work for you and which simply don't.

## 28 DAYS TO TAILOR THE DIET FOR *YOUR* UNIQUE BODY CHEMISTRY

This doesn't mean that I want you to start eating all 7 high-FI foods again. That will land you right back where you started!

Corn, peanuts and sugar should stay out 95 percent of the time. You've read about how they wreak havoc in your body, and by this point, you've felt the positive benefits of eliminating them from your diet, so why go back now? If you end up eating a piece of organic corn at a barbecue or having some organic peanut butter on a slice of apple every now and then—like once a month—that's fine. But basically, let these foods go. There are healthier choices out there. Artificial sweeteners are so bad for you that I don't want you consuming them at all. Ever. They have no place in a healthy diet. Sugar should always be kept to a minimum: 2 ounces of dark chocolate or three bites of something sweet when it is really, really worth it (and no more than 1 or 2 times per week). Remember, there are great natural sweetener options out there, including xylitol and stevia.

Cycle 2 gives you the chance to create your own individualized diet plan.

The foods we're testing in Cycle 2 include two potentially healthy foods (eggs and dairy) and two potentially unhealthy foods (soy and gluten). Why are we testing soy and gluten if I don't want you relying on them? Basically, we need to find out if you should be hypervigilant about keeping them out 100 percent of the time or just ordinarily vigilant and keeping them out 95 percent of the time.

So we're taking four foods—gluten, soy, eggs and dairy—and we're going to find out whether your system can tolerate them. Each week, you'll eat one challenge food for 4 days and then stop eating it for the next 3. If you stay symptom-free and continue to feel terrific, you're good to go. For the time being, you can have limited quantities of that food in your diet. (I will want you to challenge these foods out once a year to make sure you're still tolerating them well, but we'll get to that in Cycle 3.)

However, if you have symptoms, feel uncomfortable or just don't enjoy these foods any more, you will continue to leave them out of your diet. You always have the option of checking in 3, 6 or 9 months later to give them another try.

Remember how I told you that your body wasn't a bank account but a chemistry lab? I want you to think of Cycle 2 as a science experiment.

You're going to find out exactly what your body can handle—and what it can't. The result will be an individualized diet perfectly tailored to your own unique body chemistry.

What I love about Cycle 2 is that it gives you the chance to create your own individualized diet plan, the one that is perfectly attuned to where your body is at this point in your life. We are all so different, and we all change so much throughout the years. Why shouldn't our diets be individualized and change along with us?

 ## UNDERSTANDING CYCLE 2

Don't worry, I'm going to give you precise instructions for how to conduct Cycle 2, complete with recipes for each of the 4 days you challenge foods back in. You'll know exactly what to do.

But before you get started, I want to be sure you understand what Cycle 2 is and what it isn't. I've seen lots of clients who treat Cycle 2 as a chance to go wild and pig out on the forbidden foods they've been avoiding for 3 weeks. Sorry, folks, that just won't work. The only way to be successful on Cycle 2 is to follow every detail of the program exactly as I lay it out, or you're not going to get the results you want.

Whenever I think about getting in the right frame of mind for Cycle 2, I think of my client Taylor. She was so psyched to be starting this cycle! Although the first few days of Cycle 1 were tough for her, she ended the 3 weeks feeling absolutely terrific. She had successfully lost 10 pounds and was excited to keep going until she dropped the other 25 pounds that she wanted to get rid of. Her skin had cleared up, her hair was in great shape, and she felt more energized, focused and optimistic than she had in years.

Now we were up to Cycle 2, and Taylor was already planning all the great meals she expected to have. "It's going to taste so good to have macaroni and cheese again," she said excitedly. "And I'm going to make a big tofu stir-fry, and I can't wait to have omelets for breakfast again, with rye toast . . . and maybe I can even have some ice cream, as a special treat?"

I didn't know whether to laugh or cry. "Taylor, how do you feel now?" I asked.

"Terrific!" she said promptly. "It's not just the weight. I *feel* lighter. Clearer. Happier. For the first time in a long time, my body feels like *me* again."

"Great," I said. "And how do you think it got that way?"

We were on the phone, so I couldn't see Taylor's face, but when she took a few minutes to answer me, I could imagine her puzzled look.

"Well, obviously I dropped all these high-FI foods that were so bad for me," she finally said. "But I thought this was the cycle where we put them all back in?"

Now I did laugh.

"Taylor," I said, "we took them out because they were making you sick. What do you think is going to happen if we put them back in?"

"Ummm . . . they'll make me sick again? But I thought I only had to take them out for 3 weeks?"

"Okay, Taylor, here's the deal. First, we are never having you load up your diet with things that aren't good for you. Maybe when we get to Cycle 3, you can have a few bites of something you wouldn't normally eat, every few weeks or so, but we are not having you go back to eating junk that is just going to put on the pounds, sap your energy and start your symptoms back up again."

Cycle 2, I told her, was not about indulging. Dairy on Cycle 2 does not mean ice cream, and gluten does not mean white flour. Instead, Cycle 2 is all about finding out which *healthy* foods you can tolerate and which ones you can't.

"Think of Cycle 2 as a science experiment," I told her. "We took out the foods that were making you sick. We got you healthy, and now we're going to find out whether you can tolerate these foods in small amounts. But we are sticking to the *healthiest* versions of these foods, and we are still trying them in small amounts."

> Cycle 2 is about finding out which *healthy* foods you can tolerate and which ones you can't.

Taylor was quiet for another minute or two. Then she laughed. "Okay," she said. "I get it. There just aren't any shortcuts. I guess if I want to keep feeling this way and looking this way, I should just keep eating this way. Because this is the way that works."

## YOUR 4-WEEK PLAN

### WEEK 1: TEST THE GLUTEN

- Monday to Thursday, add 1 meal that includes gluten to your meal plan. (See recipes on pages 284-285.)
- Friday to Sunday, go back to your gluten-free diet.
- Track your symptoms every day using the symptoms checklist from my website at www.thevirgindiet.com/symptomschecklist.
- Continue to have at least one Virgin Diet Shake each day, stay hydrated and follow the Golden Rules of Meal Timing.

## WEEK 2: TEST THE SOY

- Monday to Thursday, add 1 meal that includes soy to your meal plan. (See recipes on pages 286–287.)
- Friday to Sunday, go back to your soy-free diet.
- Track your symptoms every day using the symptoms checklist from my website at www.thevirgindiet.com/symptomschecklist.
- Continue to have at least one Virgin Diet Shake each day, stay hydrated and follow the Golden Rules of Meal Timing.

## WEEK 3: TEST THE EGGS

- Monday to Thursday, add 1 meal that includes eggs to your meal plan. (See recipes on pages 287–288.)
- Friday to Sunday, go back to your egg-free diet.
- Track your symptoms every day using the symptoms checklist from my website at www.thevirgindiet.com/symptomschecklist.
- Continue to have at least one Virgin Diet Shake each day, stay hydrated and follow the Golden Rules of Meal Timing.

## WEEK 4: TEST THE DAIRY

- Monday to Thursday, add 1 meal that includes dairy to your meal plan. (See recipes on pages 289–290.)

- Friday to Sunday, go back to your dairy-free diet.

- Track your symptoms every day using the symptoms checklist from my website at www.thevirgindiet.com/symptomschecklist.

- Continue to have at least one Virgin Diet Shake each day, stay hydrated and follow the Golden Rules of Meal Timing.

Even if you discover that you can tolerate gluten, soy or eggs, *do not* add them back into your diet during the other three challenge weeks. Your goal is to keep your diet free of high-FI foods *except* for the one you are testing. Each week you are testing only *one* high-FI food. If you don't keep all of them out except for the one you're testing, it will be very hard to evaluate your results. During Cycle 2, we want to give your body only small changes to react to. Adding in too many foods at the same time will confuse your body and make it harder for you to find out what you can and cannot tolerate.

I've provided healthy soy, gluten, egg and dairy recipes for Cycle 2 in Chapter 12.

> Adding in too many foods at the same time will make it harder for you to find out what you can and cannot tolerate.

## SPOTTING FOOD INTOLERANCE

In Chapter 2, I told you to start keeping a food journal and record your symptoms. Now I want you to rate them again each day.

I can't stress too strongly how important this is. Remember, food sensitivities are sneaky. We don't know how intensely they'll strike or how soon. If you eat a food 4 days in a row, you might feel something immediately, you might have symptoms 72 hours after the first bite or you might not notice anything for a whole 7 days. That's why I have you reintroduce a food for 4 days and then take 3 days off before starting the next food. I don't want you to get confused.

**Food sensitivities are sneaky.**

Basically, the only way to find out whether you can tolerate a food is to track your symptoms. If you don't have any symptoms, you're probably fine to keep eating eggs and/or dairy, at least in healthy versions and in small quantities. You're probably also fine to allow a little gluten and soy to sneak in from time to time—but it shouldn't make up more than 5 percent of your diet long term.

If you have symptoms, though, that's your body telling you no, or at least not yet. And if you keep eating a food despite having symptoms, I can tell you what is almost certainly going to happen: your symptoms will get worse, and the lost pounds will come back.

Remember, eating a food to which you react badly is potentially creating an immune reaction. This produces immune complexes that spark inflammation, which in turn create symptoms and weight gain. If you keep eating a food that you can't tolerate, your inflammation increases, your symptoms intensify, you start craving the very food that's hurting you—and your weight continues to rise.

Now, let's look at what happens once you stop eating a food that used to give you trouble. Before, your body was full of antibodies that your immune system created over time to protect you from those specific foods. But when you stop eating those foods, those antibodies gradually disappear. So even one small bite might be enough to give you a powerful reaction. Certainly, after eating the food for 4 days in a row, you're going to see symptoms if you have any intolerance at all.

There's another possibility. You might be fine with the food in small quantities, say, if you eat it for a day or two. But then, if you eat that food day after day, you might have gas, bloating and all the other symptoms. Then you start to create more of those antibodies, and that's when your body starts to create an immune attack.

This is why I recommend that you rotate eggs and/or dairy into your diet only every fourth day, or at most every other day, depending on how you responded to the challenge. Not eating reactive foods every day prevents the buildup of the immune complexes and the antibodies that your body has so much trouble getting rid of.

## WHY THE TIMING MATTERS

Quite often you will have a far more pronounced response to your problem foods now that your body has had a chance to heal and you have significantly reduced the antibodies. If you notice a severe reaction right away, you have your answer and do not need to keep challenging the food. You can see that this food isn't working for you right now, but if you give your body at least 3 to 6 months to heal, you might be able to tolerate it in the future.

This is what happened to me with eggs. The first time I rechallenged them, I was doubled over with stomach cramps. However, 6 months later, I found that I could tolerate them in small amounts rotated every 4 days or so into my diet.

If you notice mild symptoms over the next 24 to 72 hours, I would again pull the food out and rechallenge in another 3 to 6 months. I have found that when I eat gluten, my fingers are swollen the next day. Although this isn't incapacitating, I know that it means that gluten is creating an inflammatory response that will not be good for my body on a regular basis.

If you notice mild symptoms on the fourth day, then you can rotate this food into your diet every 4 days. The reason I chose 4 days here is because that is typically how long it takes for the antibodies to start building up. So if you rotate a food that you are showing a reaction to only after consuming it for 4 days straight, you should be fine.

Finally, if you show no reaction, especially to eggs and/or dairy, then these are foods that you can work into your diet. But again, rotate them in so you are not eating them every single day. Every second or third day is fine. If you don't react to gluten or soy, you can have some occasionally, but please don't make either food a mainstay of your diet. Not reacting to these foods means that you don't have to be hypervigilant about keeping them out. If you have the occasional piece of sourdough bread or miso soup, you will be fine.

## REINTRODUCTION RECIPES

I've provided healthy soy, gluten, egg and dairy recipes for Cycle 2 in Chapter 12—just turn to pages 261–291.

# FREQUENTLY ASKED QUESTIONS

### Q: Will I still lose weight on Cycle 2?

A: If you don't react to any of the four rechallenges, then yes, you should. Consuming a food that you can't tolerate will stall your weight loss, and this is exactly what we need to find out in Cycle 2: which foods will stall your weight loss. Once you are eating only the foods that you can tolerate, your weight loss should return to its optimal rate.

### Q: On Cycle 2, can I just start eating the foods I dropped on Cycle 1?

A: No way. I've created a very specific plan for how to reintroduce each food, and I've given you recipes and a meal plan to help you conduct this "science experiment" in exactly the right way. You need to follow the plan to find out exactly how these high-FI foods affect you.

### Q: How will I know if I can tolerate a food or not?

A: Don't worry, you'll know! Usually, if people react badly, their symptoms are through the roof almost immediately, and as a result, they don't even *want* the food any more. However, the symptoms are sometimes more delayed or more subtle. That's why I want you to track your symptoms every day.

### Q: What happens if I react badly to a food on Cycle 2?

A: You might decide to let that food go for life, or you might repeat Cycle 2 in 3, 6 or 12 months. Possibly, foods that you can't tolerate now will become easier to handle once your system has further healed.

## Q: Once I know I can tolerate a food, can I just keep it in my diet?

A: Not yet. Even if you find out during week 1 that you can tolerate gluten, for example, I want you to stay gluten-free for the rest of the month. I don't want you to introduce soy, dairy or eggs while you are also eating gluten. I want to keep your diet as low-FI as possible while you are introducing each new high-FI food.

## Q: What about *after* Cycle 2? If I can tolerate a food, can I just keep it in my diet?

A: That depends. If you notice a symptom in the first day, then that's not a food that you should be eating. You can rechallenge it again in 3 months if you want. If you notice a symptom by the fourth day, you can put that food into your diet every fourth day—not any more often, or you might start reacting more intensely. If you don't notice any symptoms, then sure, enjoy! I still don't want you to eat eggs or dairy every day because you could start to build up an immune response that will lead to reactivity, but every other day should be fine. And of course, no matter what happens, I don't want you building a meal around soy or gluten. We are only testing those to find out whether they stay out 100 percent or 95 percent.

## ▍ HEALTHY CHOICES ONLY, PLEASE!

As I told Taylor, for each of the four rechallenge weeks, you want the healthiest versions of each food that you can find. For gluten, you want to choose whole grains only, so go for whole-wheat pasta and whole-grain pita when the recipes call for that. And long term, seek out grains that have been sprouted. Sprouting grains reduces the phytic acid, which is an antinutrient that interferes with the absorption of minerals. If you sprout your grains, you might even discover that you can handle them just fine. However, during this time, I want you to challenge with more common food choices.

Likewise, when you add soy, you want the healthiest version you can find, so I want you to seek out organic soy. I am allowing a little miso, along with tofu and veggie burgers. If you find that you don't react to soy, then ideally limit your intake long term to organic, fermented choices and, again, keep this to 5 percent of your overall diet.

During your egg week, go for the organic eggs only. If you can get into a farmer's cooperative or collective, that would be much better because then you can be sure that your eggs came from healthy chickens.

Dairy week is all about the healthy choices. We're having Greek yogurt, mozzarella or cottage cheese—not ice cream, whipped cream or other foods that aren't good for us for other reasons. Also, be sure to choose organic and preferably the low-fat version. Stay away from the nonfat versions, though, because these often have other additives to make up for the lost fat. If you can't find low-fat, then I would prefer that you go for full fat. Stick with cow's milk here because you might handle sheep's or goat's milk products differently. If you're okay with cow's milk, then sheep's and goat's milk products should be fine. If you're not okay with cow's milk, do a separate challenge with sheep's and goat's milk because you might be able to handle those. (For more on sheep's and goat's milk, see Chapter 5.)

If you decide to add eggs and dairy back into your diet, stick with the healthy choices, please! Otherwise, you're just giving yourself permission to eat bad foods that will set you up for symptoms and put back on the weight you worked so hard to lose. And if eating healthy versions of eggs and dairy causes you to start craving the unhealthy versions, you might consider pulling them out completely.

#  ARE YOU AN OUTLIER?

After the first few days of Cycle 1, you should feel remarkably better. If you don't, I want you to dig deeper. Don't assume that this program doesn't work.

First, check to make sure that you pulled out all the high-FI foods 100 percent. Remember my story about the tacks? It's not enough to remove three of the four tacks. Your butt is still going to hurt when you sit down.

Next, consider the possibility that you're intolerant to some other foods. We've started with the top 7 high-FI foods—the ones most likely to provoke sensitivities or create inflammatory responses—but you might also have trouble with the second tier: shellfish, tree nuts, citrus and strawberries. So you might give yourself a 3-week period to drop those completely from your diet and see what happens.

Finally, you might be one of those outliers who have unique responses to a particular food. If you're still having symptoms or struggling with losing weight, find a functional medical practitioner and get yourself tested for IgG food sensitivities. It's a very simple test: they take one tiny drop of your blood and send it off to a lab. In about 10 days, you'll get a complete reading on your degree of sensitivity to a whole panel of foods. (See the Resources section on my website for suggestions on how to find such a practitioner.)

Remember, though, IgG food sensitivities only show one type of reaction to food, so they won't tell you the whole story. The best test of all is to pull out the most common foods and gauge how you feel. Only use a lab test as a follow-up if you haven't made the progress you should have or if you are still struggling with symptoms.

# LOOKING TO YOUR GUT FOR THE ANSWERS

What if your test shows that you don't have any IgG sensitivities, but you still have symptoms? Then you might have some other gastrointestinal issues that need to be addressed. You may have problems with your *biofilm,* the organisms that might have taken up residence on your intestinal lining.

- **Small intestine bacterial overgrowth.** If you still have gas and bloating that gets worse throughout the day, consider this condition, in which the bad bacteria in your intestines has gotten out of control. You're always going to have some bad bacteria in your system, but your goal is to have more of the good bacteria in there. If the balance tips the wrong way, that bad bacteria extracts more calories from the food you eat and stores it as fat. It can push things out of control. Find a functional medical practitioner or naturopath to help you fix this problem.

- **Yeast overgrowth.** This is a similar problem to small intestine bacterial overgrowth—yeast that grows throughout your gastrointestinal tract. Yeast overgrowth can set up sugar cravings that feel nearly uncontrollable, so you might want to check this out as well.

- **Parasites.** These can cause a lot of trouble. If you've traveled to Latin America, Asia or Africa or recently gone camping, your chances of picking up parasites is greater than normal. See a doctor who can help you detect and eliminate them.

- **Poor digestion.** Eating too fast or eating while stressed can harm your digestion even if you don't have specific food intolerances. You might also be lacking digestive enzymes or be low in stomach acid. Try taking a comprehensive digestive enzyme or work with a specialist to diagnose and solve the problem.

> **Your gut determines so much of your health.**

Your gut determines so much of your health. It all starts there. When you feel gassy and bloated, it ruins every bit of your day. So please, if you still feel that way, consider your gut biofilm. What we did over the last couple weeks was a great start toward a healthier biofilm. We took out the things that would feed yeast and bad bacteria. But if you are still having problems, you might want to consider working with a practitioner who can suggest supplements to help you with any area in which you have an issue. (See the Resources section on my website.)

## I'M INTOLERANT—NOW WHAT?

I know it can be tough discovering that your favorite foods are not good for you. Sometimes the truth hurts. But in the end, it's always better to know.

Believe me, I've been there. I can rotate dairy into my diet, but I get mucous right away and acne 2 days later. It never fails. I always think, *Do I want a zit or not? Is it worth it or not?* Greek-style yogurt is one of my most favorite things on the planet, and I used to love that inch of foamy milk on my cafè Americano. It's the same with eggs. If I eat eggs that are clean, I can handle them every once in a while. If they're not, they hurt me. I get gassy and bloated, and my stomach aches like you wouldn't believe. Gluten tends to swell my fingers. If I eat it at dinner, the next day I wake up and can feel it when I bend my fingers. I can't tolerate gluten, and I've learned to live with it.

Your experiences with these high-FI foods might be just like mine, or they might be completely different. The only way to know is to go through Cycle 2. Once you know the truth, you can act on it. You'll be amazed at how powerful that makes you feel.

# HOW THE VIRGIN DIET WORKED FOR ME

Ursula Lesic
Age 45

Allison Park,
Pennsylvania

**Height:**
5'1"

**Starting Weight:**
190 pounds

**Waist:** 39"
**Hips:** 48"

**Current Weight:**
130 pounds

**Waist:** 30"
**Hips:** 38"

**Lost:** 60 pounds

I was only 5'1", but I weighed in at 190 pounds. I was under lots of stress as a caregiver for my mom and as a manager in corporate America, and I just couldn't take the weight off. I tried low-calorie, low-fat, eating grapefruits before a meal and drinking glasses and glasses of water. Nothing worked until I started working with JJ and gave up sugar and gluten.

All of a sudden, my scale went down by a half pound each day, plus once a week, I would drop another 2 pounds overnight. I came out of my brain fog and moodiness and had tons of energy. That was the energy I needed to begin to exercise to tone and build muscle. Now, at age 45, I am more healthy and vibrant than I was in my 20s.

# CYCLE 3: THE VIRGIN DIET FOR LIFE

**10**

First of all, congratulations! You have completed Cycles 1 and 2 of the Virgin Diet, which in my opinion is a *huge* achievement. Look around you. So many people are not taking care of themselves. They are eating all the wrong foods, gaining weight and feeling sick. But that is not you! You cared enough about yourself and the people who love you to complete the first 7 weeks of the Virgin Diet, and now you are reaping the rewards.

I know it hasn't always been easy, but you have so much to be proud of! So, for your very first action in Cycle 3, I want you to go out and give yourself a huge reward, something that matches the big achievement that you have just accomplished.

> You have so much to be proud of!

Now, I don't want that reward to be a food reward. Part of Cycle 3—which is basically the rest of your life—is going to involve building in other kinds of rewards to keep you happy with your new body, glowing with your new health and motivated to keep up this healthy new way of eating for life.

I can hear some of you thinking, *Hmmmm. A nonfood reward. What might that be?*

I know where you're coming from. We can get so focused on using food as our reward system that we forget all the other fabulous ways to give ourselves special treats. But you know what? If you don't start building a system of nonfood rewards into your regular life—not just on holidays or vacations, but as part of your daily and weekly routine—you are not going to make it on the Virgin Diet. If the only sweetness in your day comes from sugar, and the primary pleasure in your life comes from chocolate, there is just no way that you are going to avoid sugar and stick to 2 ounces of dark chocolate (which you *are* allowed!).

Most diets focus on what you have to take out. That's why most of them don't work so well. So let's start focusing on what you are going to put in. Here are some ideas for your very first Virgin Diet reward.

- **A manicure or a pedicure at your favorite salon.** If you don't have a favorite salon, find one! For an extra reward, ask for the 15-minute leg massage that most salons offer with the spa pedicure. Mmmmm…

- **A facial.** These are great when you've been doing the Virgin Diet because your skin is already in such good shape. Guys, you know you can have one, too, right?

- **A massage.** If you are missing quality time with your significant other, you might even splurge on a couples' massage.

- **Some lingerie or a great new outfit that shows off your fabulous new body.** Don't make the mistake of waiting until you've hit your ideal weight to start dressing for the new you. If you can't enjoy your improvements along the way, how are you going to stay motivated to keep getting better?

- **A long, fragrant bath with some new foaming bubble bath, silky bath oil or exotic bath gel.** Get yourself a new loofah or a fresh plastic scrubber so you can exfoliate in style. Maybe throw in a new flavor of body butter or moisturizer to celebrate your glowing skin after the bath.

- **An adventure.** Visit a part of your city that you've never seen, take a drive to a new part of your county or hop on a bus or train to a neighboring town. Wander through some new streets or stroll through some new countryside. Go solo or take a friend or loved one who you've been meaning to spend quality time with.

- **A time-out.** Find a quiet spot that brings you peace—in your home, a neighborhood coffee shop, a local park or any other place that you enjoy—and just zone out for a little while. Take a book or a magazine, put on some headphones with your favorite music, sip a cup of herbal tea or fresh-brewed coffee and give yourself a minivacation from all the demands of your life.

Does this list give you some more ideas for rewards, treats and other pleasures? That's terrific! I want you to start keeping a list, right now, of nonfood rewards and pleasures. Start to build those into your weekly and monthly routine. In this chapter, we'll also look at exercise, stress release and ways to stay motivated because studies have shown that the techniques that help you *maintain* a healthy weight are actually quite different from the approach you need to *lose* weight. If you still have more weight to lose to reach your ideal body composition, we will address this as well. So basically, in this chapter, I'll make sure your motivational maintenance tool kit is fully stocked. I'll tell you everything you need to know about eating healthy and maintaining the Virgin Diet for the rest of your life.

## MAINTAINING THE VIRGIN DIET FOR LIFE IN CYCLE 3

- Continue assembling meals as before, using the Virgin Diet Plate and focusing on clean, lean protein; healthy fats; high-fiber, low-glycemic carbs; and nonstarchy vegetables.

- At least 95 percent of the time, avoid sugar, artificial sweeteners, gluten, corn, soy and peanuts.

- If you can tolerate them, include healthy forms of eggs and dairy based on how you did in Cycle 2: If you had no reaction, you can eat them every other day. If you had a reaction by the fourth day, you can eat them every 4 days. If you reacted immediately, leave them out for at least 3 months.

- Follow the Golden Rules of Meal Timing (see pages 172–173).

- Substitute 1 meal each day with a Virgin Diet Shake (see page 170).

- Stay hydrated.

- Move more and do real exercise (see pages 225–235).

- Get 7 to 9 hours of high-quality sleep each night.

- Devote at least 15 minutes per day to your own personal bliss.

## PLANNING: THE KEY TO YOUR SUCCESS

Have you ever heard the old saying "When you fail to plan, you plan to fail"? In my experience, that is true in every area of your life—and nowhere more than when it comes to maintaining a healthy weight. The rates of weight regain after a typical diet are anywhere from 50 to

95 percent depending on the research being cited.[29, 30] And friends, we will not be part of those statistics, deal?

Let's face it, when you're starting a new diet, even a challenging one, you have lots of motivation to follow the program. On the Virgin Diet, you might have had trouble pulling out some of your standby foods or subbing in healthy choices for unhealthy ones, but there's something about the newness of it all that can keep you going. It's like dating an exciting new person: you don't necessarily know where things are going, but you're willing to put in that extra effort to dress nicely, stay groomed and figure out fun things to do together.

Then, you get into a steady relationship or even get married, and suddenly, all of that effort goes out the window. Now you don't always bother to shave, dress up or plan romantic evenings. Now you're just hanging out in your sweats in front of the TV. Then you wonder where the magic has gone.

It's the same thing with the Virgin Diet. As we just saw, you need to plan in some rewards to keep things new and fresh. But you also need to plan for the daily stuff because this is something that you're going to be doing for life. So let's figure out how.

- **Are you bringing food to work each day so you can eat healthy and avoid the vending machine or coffee bar?** How do you build in time to get that food together every single day so you're never tempted to skip when you're running late? Maybe there's a way you can get everything together Sunday night, or maybe you can combine watching a favorite TV program with putting together the next day's food. Think about it. Build it in.

- **What about shopping? When have you built that into your schedule?** How can you make sure to never run out of the things you need to stay on the program? If you've got to drive across town to find the coconut milk, how do you make sure to allow that time so you don't end up just throwing in some regular milk from the convenience store? Is there a way that you can order some things you need online? Is there a friend or neighbor or someone at work who is also doing the Virgin Diet who can take turns with you in getting some of the hard-to-find items? Get creative. There are always new ways to solve problems once you're open to finding them.

- **Are there particular pitfalls that you _know_ are going to be tough for you: Sunday family dinners, holiday parties or a day at the amusement park with your kids?** These kinds of things are never total surprises—you pretty much know they're going to happen sometime. What can you do now to get ready for them when they do? One of my clients keeps a stash of turkey jerky, raw nuts and apples on hand. If she finds out that she's going to be away from home all day, she throws some of her high-protein snacks into some zip-lock plastic bags and grabs an apple. Now she's set, no matter what happens that day. Because she plans ahead and keeps everything well stocked at home, she never has to worry about missing a meal or eating the wrong foods on the road.

## DON'T SKIP THE SHAKES!

I am a huge fan of replacing 1 meal per day with a Virgin Diet Shake— and when you're traveling, rushed or have just found yourself slipping, I am happy to see you replace 2 meals with shakes.

Why? Because multiple studies have shown that people who replace 1 meal per day with a shake lose more weight and keep it off. And still more studies have shown that people who incorporate protein into their diets throughout the day also maintain their weight more easily. Virgin Diet Shakes are part of the balanced approach that keeps you feeling full and nourished all day.

 ## IF YOU ENJOY A DRINK NOW AND THEN...

When you get to Cycle 3, you can enjoy a glass of red wine, even every day if you would like. I know you've heard that alcohol can help reduce your risk of heart disease. It can, but only in the right amounts: one glass max for women and two for men. In fact, studies have shown that people who drink a glass of red wine each day are thinner than people who don't. I think it's probably because it helps them reduce stress. Also, they are probably not having dessert. They are having wine.

Pinot noir has the highest resveratrol content. Resveratrol is an amazing antioxidant and is also anti-inflammatory. It's also been found to switch on the gene that helps slow down the aging process. Drink it with my blessing in Cycle 3—in the right quantity.

Because red wine is full of antioxidants and other healthy ingredients, I prefer it over white. But white wine and even champagne are also okay in moderation.

As for beer, they don't call it a beer belly for nothing. I wonder if the reason beer does this so much is because it contains gluten. You can buy gluten-free beer now, and when you reach Cycle 3, you might be able to tolerate a little gluten. Avoid all types of beer in Cycles 1 and 2 and perhaps treat yourself to one gluten-free beer per week in Cycle 3.

If you have beer, choose dark beers. They are rich in *Saccharomyces boulardii,* which helps reduce bacterial overgrowth; raises secretory IgA, which drives your major gut immune system; and may help prevent yeast overgrowth. Dark beer is a great probiotic, too.

Mixed drinks are where you can get in trouble because they are often full of sugar and easy to suck down. In general, I'd like you to stay away from them, although a bloody Mary is fine. Tequila is another exception, which you can also have every week or so. But only one shot and not in a sugary mix, which is what you'll get in most margaritas. Drink it straight or try the delicious mixture that I invented myself and got a Chicago barman to mix up for me (see page 291 for the recipe).

Of course, if you aren't currently an imbiber, I don't recommend starting! Women's risk of breast cancer increases with alcohol intake, so be careful. One glass of wine is fine. More than that is a problem.

## THE THREE-BITE RULE

One of the great joys of Cycle 3 is that you get to splurge on forbidden foods 5 percent of the time, and yes, that does include dessert. So if you are looking forward to a few bites of birthday cake or a taste of your sister-in-law's famous cornbread stuffing, you will get your chance! But I don't want you taking advantage of this rule, or pretty soon you'll have undone all the good work you just spent the last 7 weeks on. The safest way to indulge in Cycle 3 is to follow the three-bite rule: once or twice a week, you can have *three* bites of something you otherwise wouldn't eat as long as it isn't something to which you react badly. If you're having more than three bites more than twice a week, you've passed the 5 percent mark. And remember, if you had an extreme reaction to one of the challenge foods in Cycle 2, you will not want to take even three bites of it.

Now, when I say three bites, I don't mean truck driver bites! I mean three polite bites, the kind you'd have if you were eating in front of an audience on national TV.

Let's say you are out somewhere. They have something amazing. It is not something that you react to. Here are the rules:

1. Make sure it's really, really worth it. Why waste your indulgence on fat-free angel food cake or a kid's sugary ice cream confection? Save this for something fabulous!

2. If possible, share with someone who has a faster fork. If I'm going to have dessert, I have it with my mother, who can plow through something sweet faster than anyone I've ever seen. The only ones who rival her are my kids!

3. If you're going solo, pull out the three bites before you start eating and then get rid of the rest. Put ketchup on top of it. Have the waiter take it away. Don't just throw it in the trash. We all saw what happened on that *Seinfeld* episode: you can still dig it out! Set yourself up for success by getting rid of the extra food *before* you take your first bite.

4. The whole reason for this rule is to give yourself a guilt-free treat. Give yourself permission to enjoy this, and then don't beat yourself up. *Do not* use this as a reason to go on a guilt-fueled binge. You haven't done anything wrong!

5. If you need to put closure on the incident, have a mint or brush your teeth.

# THE IMPORTANCE OF RECHALLENGING

By this point, you've come to see that health is a dynamic process. You can create leaky gut and then heal it. You can tolerate something for a while and then build up immune complexes that set up intolerance. You can eat something when your life is going well and then develop problems under stress. Our bodies are always changing, just as our lives are. You have to be prepared for this.

I'm so proud of you for making it to Cycle 3! But I don't want you to assume that you're done and that there is nothing more to discover about your health. You might be able to tolerate dairy or eggs now, but that doesn't mean you can do so next year—or vice versa. So, I recommend moving through Cycles 1, 2 and 3 once a year, every year, for the rest of your life. You can choose whichever time of year works best for you, but I often find this works well as a "new year, new you" program, in the spring to get ready for summer or in the fall after too much summer vacation. If you have developed some food intolerances, you might see rapid fat loss again in Cycle 1. And if you have some weight to lose, focusing on your food quality and quantity and going back to journaling is definitely going to help.

When you go back through the cycles, you may have some surprises, which might possibly work both ways. Something you could never eat turns into a food you tolerate. Something you could always eat turns into a food you can't tolerate. This isn't me trying to trip you up, this is the way your body works. I'm trying to set you up for success by sharing this knowledge with you and encouraging you to take charge of your own health. If you'd rather spend the money, you can go to a functional doctor or naturopath and get tested for food sensitivities once a year. But I'd rather you do this program because then you are most closely in touch with your own body and your own responses. Practitioners will mainly test you for IgG sensitivies, but there are other ways that your body might react poorly to food. That's why I find that the very best test is the elimination diet. The sense of power you get from doing that will spill over into the rest of your life. I promise you, there is nothing like it.

---

## THE VIRGIN DIET: THE LIFETIME PROGRAM

- At least 95 percent of the time, avoid sugar, fruit juices and high-glycemic juices, corn, soy and peanuts. Follow the "three *polite* bites" rule the other 5 percent of the time. Avoid artificial sweeteners 100 percent of the time.

- If you can tolerate them, include healthy forms of eggs and dairy based on how you did in Cycle 2: If you had no reaction, you can eat them every other day. If you had a reaction by the fourth day, you can eat them every 4 days. If you reacted immediately, leave them out for at least 3 months.

- Once every 3 months, feel free to rechallenge the foods you cannot tolerate. Go back to Chapter 9 and repeat any or all of the gluten, soy, egg or dairy challenges. *This is optional.*

- Once every 12 months, go back to Chapter 8 and repeat the 21 days of the Virgin Diet, then move on to Chapter 9 and rechallenge any or all of the 4 foods. *This is a necessity. You must do it every year.*

---

I WASN'T KIDDING: MODERATION CAN MAKE YOU FAT

A recent study showed that people at a healthy weight who ate moderately were likely to gain 10 pounds in 10 years. Just 1 pound per year can make the difference between zipping up your jeans and having to buy a new pair—or the difference between feeling old, overweight and unattractive versus facing middle age with lots of vitality, sparkle and confidence in your fit and glowing body.

> I have to work hard at staying in shape and staying on the program, just like you do.

I am not just saying this to you, I am saying it to myself. Believe it or not, I have to work hard at staying in shape and staying on the program, just like you do. There was a time in my life when I found that I had gained 10 pounds, my waistline had thickened, my skin was breaking out and I felt foggy and under par. Slowly but surely, I was feeling the effects of my beloved whey shakes, goat cheese omelets, sourdough bread and that inch of foamy milk on my cafè Americano. When I cut out eggs, dairy and gluten, the weight came off, my skin cleared up and my mental sharpness returned. I had learned my lesson. Now I want to share it with you. As long as I stay on the program, I never have to think about my weight. It is so liberating to never have to worry about my weight or if my pants are going to zip up. After all, weight loss shouldn't be a hobby.

So, how do we guard against the dangers of moderation? Here are the tips I've figured out for myself. I know they will work for you, too.

- **Weigh and measure yourself once a week.** We always want to get on the scale when we know we're in great shape and avoid it when we've slipped. Nope. That is setting yourself up for failure, and I want you to set yourself up for success. Weigh in weekly—pick the same time of day so the figure is meaningful—and write down the weight in your food journal. Compare the number with your last three weights. Are you staying the same, going down or going up? Be honest—and take action. (For an easy measurement record you can use to track your weight and measurements, go to www.thevirgindiet.com/weighttracker.

- **Write it down.** You don't have to keep a food journal in Cycle 3 the way you did in Cycles 1 and 2, but I can tell you that when I know I've slipped—when I've eaten more than three polite bites of something or indulged in a food that I know I can't tolerate—I get out the journal that night and track myself for the next week. I want to know if I have got symptoms creeping in, and I want to take action if I do. If you feel like you're falling off the food wagon or if you notice symptoms—acne, rosacea, gas, bloating, indigestion, fatigue, mental fog or crankiness—go back to journaling. Clean up your diet. Cut out dairy, eggs, gluten and soy for a couple weeks. Make sure you're staying hydrated. Stick extra closely to the Golden Rules of Meal Timing. Be vigilant about your daily shake and about your meal assembly with all the right ingredients.

- **Be accountable to someone.** Hire a coach, join an online support group or get a friend to become your accountability buddy. You need someone or some group that will hold you to your commitment. I do, you do, we all do.

- **Keep your eye on the prize.** Continue to up-level your inspired goals to keep you motivated and on the straight and narrow.

- **Get at least 7 to 9 hours of good sleep each night.** Be aware that suboptimal sleep—either not enough or not under the right conditions—can totally sabotage your weight, not to mention the rest of your health. This isn't just a matter of "it would be nice if . . . ." Sleep is essential. *Insufficient sleep will make you fat.*

 ## MINDFUL EATING

Here's the great thing: you can make tiny shifts that you don't even notice to help you eat and drink less. Although I want you drinking lots of water when you're not eating, remember that you need to restrict fluids while you eat.

Here is something that I do at my house. I use small, pretty plates, and I insist that everyone sit down to eat. I have two boys, so there was basically a frat house in my kitchen. I realized that with all the standing and grabbing, it was easy to overeat. When we sat down and used our pretty plates—and the nice skinny glasses that I bought to go with them—it was much easier to feel full and satisfied. When you pay attention to food, it tastes better, and your satiety goes up. If your mind is elsewhere, you keep eating mindlessly.

> When you pay attention to food, it tastes better, and your satiety goes up.

The following are a few other tips for becoming conscious of when, where, how and how much you eat. A lot of these ideas came from my hero, Brian Wansink, a Nobel Prize–winning expert in consumer behavior and nutritional science. (I've listed his fabulous book in the Sources section.)

- **Follow the Golden Rules of Meal Timing.** They'll keep you from being hungry so you're a lot less likely to feel like overeating. (See pages 172–173 if you want to review them.)

- **No bedtime snacks.** If you eat before bed, you can suppress the human growth hormone, which is key for improving your metabolism and burning fat. More important, if you ate your balanced dinner and followed your meal plan throughout the day, you're probably not hungry—just bored or thirsty. Give yourself a nonfood treat or have a glass of water. You shouldn't go to sleep with a full belly. Ghrelin—released when your stomach is empty—triggers in turn the release of the growth hormone, which helps you build muscle, speed up your metabolism and burn fat.

- **Drink 8 ounces of water in the evening.** A University of Washington study showed this will help shut down your hunger pangs.[31]

- **Stay hydrated throughout the day.** When you get hungry, ask yourself, *Is this hunger or thirst?* You'll be surprised at how often it's thirst!

- **Go for the fiber.** Remember to bring your fiber intake up slowly and to drink lots of water as you do so to give your body time to adjust. When you're eating your optimal daily fiber of 50 grams, you get a feeling of fullness that lasts for a long time.

- **Know your triggers and avoid them.** Don't have food on your shelves that will tempt you to eat between meals or overeat. If you can't buy food in small quantities (e.g., chocolate), freeze it in individual portion sizes so you have to defrost it before you eat. That way, you won't be as likely to eat on impulse.

- **Put away leftovers before you start eating.** You can't have seconds if the food is already stored in the fridge and cold before you've finished your firsts.

- **Write down *everything* you eat.** That way, you won't be nearly as tempted to cheat.

- **Put your fork down between every bite.** Nothing is better for helping you pay attention to each bite.

- **Use chopsticks.** This will also slow you down.

- **Weigh and measure to relearn portions.** Your own judgment will be out of whack for a few weeks, so use external measures until you've internalized them.

- **Dine with slow eaters.** You will tend to follow their rhythm, which means you'll stop being hungry a lot sooner.

I personally use these tips all the time, so I'm psyched to share them with you. You don't have to start them all at the same time. Try adding one each week until they all become second nature.

## IF YOU STILL WANT TO LOSE WEIGHT…

If you are not at your ideal weight yet, don't worry. If you stick to the Virgin Diet, you will find that you will continue to lose weight until you reach your ideal body composition. Just keep out sugar, corn, peanuts, gluten and soy 95 percent of the time and only eat dairy and eggs to the extent you can tolerate them based on your results in Cycle 2.

Be sure to continue journaling during this time. If you find that your weight loss stalls, be sure to incorporate the long-term strategies including burst training and resistance exercise, good sleep and stress management.

While you are actively working on weight loss, don't have even three bites of a forbidden food and limit your alcohol intake. You can also go back to two shakes a day to accelerate your weight loss.

If you are doing everything right and get "stuck," it is time to visit a functional medicine practitioner (see the Resources section on my website) to get evaluated for weight-loss resistance due to other factors, including gastrointestinal issues (small intestine bacterial overgrowth, yeast, parasites), thyroid disease, insulin or leptin resistance, toxicity and sex hormone imbalances.

 ## GET MOVING

One of the best ways that you can maintain your ideal weight—and also stay healthy, energized and fit—is to exercise. Although exercise isn't so important for losing weight, studies have shown that it is absolutely crucial for maintaining weight.[32, 33] If you've already been working out, doing cardio or moving a lot, congratulations! Keep it up or bump it up.

If you have been fairly sedentary up to this point, now is the time to get yourself in gear.

You won't necessarily go from sitting on the couch all day to achieving your ideal fitness. But you can do it gradually, through a three-step process:

1. Move more.
2. Start burst-style training.
3. Add resistance training.

## MOVE MORE

You've got to start from where you are. So no matter how little you've done up to this point, start by moving just 5 minutes per day. Take a brisk walk, walk up some stairs instead of taking the elevator, jump on your kid's bike—find some way to move even a little bit. At the end of the first week, add 5 more minutes to make it 10. Keep adding 5 minutes every week until you get up to an hour of physical activity per day.

Remember, moving is a part of life. We are supposed to move. Sometimes you have to make an effort, though, especially if you live in the suburbs or in someplace like southern California, which is where I happen to live. Hey, no one walks in southern California. We even have valet parking at the airport.

That is not acceptable to me, so thankfully I have a little dog. That helps me a lot because I have to walk her at least 15 minutes in the morning and 15 minutes at night. I make a point of parking farther away so every time I get out of my car, I move for 5 minutes before reaching my destination. I find excuses to take the stairs. If I'm in a place like Las Vegas with 40 flights of stairs, there's my exercise—stair workouts. I definitely would rather do that than pay an arm and a leg to use the fitness room.

Now, what do I mean when I say you need to get moving for an hour a day? Eventually, you'll carve out some of that time for burst-style exercise and resistance training. But if you're new to this, you'll probably want to start out by walking and finding other ways to incorporate movement and physical activity into your life. Don't worry, you don't have to take an hour walk each day. Instead, think of little places to work in 5 minutes here, 5 minutes there. Get a pedometer and find out how much you are actually moving. Then, gradually work your way up to 6,000 or more steps a day. (Did you know that a pedometer is one of the five top tools for weight loss? The other four are a journal, a scale, fiber and water, which you're already on top of! For information on where to find a pedometer, see the Resources section on my website.) The great news is that every step you take counts, so even going to the kitchen to get a glass of water gives you a boost on your way to your daily goal.

I understand that exercise of any kind might seem overwhelming at this moment. I get that. But we'll start slowly. If you start from where you are and commit to self-care and self-improvement, I really believe that you will get hooked on exercise. You will say, "What was I thinking to even *try* to live without this wonderful activity?" You'll turn into one of those people who, like me, gets a little crabby when they don't exercise. You'll discover this whole new world of feeling energized and capable and fit.

## Using a Pedometer, Step by Step

A pedometer is a great gadget that has the potential to motivate you to increase your daily activity by counting the steps you take throughout the day. A pedometer makes it easy for you to work up to your goal of 1 hour of moving each day. The great news here is that everything counts, so your resistance training, your burst training and your daily movement all contribute to your daily hour of movement. Some days you may just get in this hour through your daily life, by taking the stairs, parking farther away, running errands on foot or taking a nice, long walk. Other days you may do so much exercise that you don't even need to take the stairs or park farther away (but I encourage you to do so anyway, as it is a habit that will serve you well).

I am assuming that your average walking pace is about 3 mph which means that 10 minutes of walking equals 1,000 steps. Since I want you to do 60 minutes of total movement daily, that means you need to accumulate 6,000 steps. Again, everything counts!

Remember to track your steps and your walking time in your daily journal because what you measure, you can improve.

*Note:* The steps you collect on your pedometer count into your daily hour of movement but are not part of your daily exercise program. I still want you to do burst-style training and then add some resistance training. Your daily exercise counts toward your daily hour of movement, but you can't *just* walk. You also have to burst and do resistance! But even if you're exercising a few times a week, I also want you to move more—and the pedometer is a great way to make sure you do it. I confess, my pedometer is the only reason I ever park farther away than I need to. I can't wait for you to get motivated, too!

## WHAT IS REAL EXERCISE?

I want you to move more, but that doesn't really count as exercise in my book. In order for something to be exercise, you have to get hot and sweaty, and it should hurt a little bit. Otherwise, you will have enormous difficulty staying at your ideal weight. The two types of exercise that will work best for keeping you fit and slim are burst-style training and resistance training.

## Burst Through Your Excess Weight!

Burst exercise has you working out in short intense bursts of 30 to 60 seconds coupled with 1 to 2 minutes of active recovery, or moving at a low intensity that allows you to catch your breath and lower your heart rate. Two easy examples of this are sprinting to burst and then walking to recover, and running up stairs to burst and then walking down them to recover. You'll do this for a total of 4 to 8 total minutes of high-intensity bursts. This will take you 20 to 30 minutes, and if you are still upright at that point, you are *not* doing this hard enough.

With bursting, you do raise stress hormones, but you raise anabolic-building hormones alongside them, counteracting the negative effects of the stress hormones. The short bursts train your body how to handle stress and recover. The repeated intense bursts raise lactic acid, which in turn raises growth hormones and supports fat burning.[34] The research is clear that the more intense the exercise, the bigger metabolic cost after you are done, which causes you to burn more calories after exercise, especially calories from fat. In fact, researchers Pacheco-Sánchez and Grunwald showed more pronounced fat loss in rats that exercised at a high intensity as compared with rats that exercised at a low intensity despite both groups performing an equivalent amount of work.[35]

So, how do you get started? Grab your cross trainers or running shoes and let's go. Warm up for a few minutes and then go all out with your workout of choice for 30 to 60 seconds. If you can go past 60 seconds, you aren't doing it hard enough. Take twice as much time to recover (1 minute of recovery if you went all out for 30 seconds, or 2 minutes of recovery if you went for 1 minute) by doing a lower intensity version of the same move or walking around. Then, repeat until you accumulate between 4 and 8 minutes of high-intensity interval bursts. If you can get to 8 minutes total, I am impressed, and if you can get past that, you probably aren't doing it hard enough. Intensity is *everything* when it comes to burst-style training.

The best way to monitor your exertion here is not by using a heart rate monitor because you will be done before the device registers how high your heart rate is. Instead, pay attention to your body. You should feel your lungs and thighs burning, and you should literally feel like you have to stop. Do this every other day and watch yourself get leaner, stronger and more energetic practically overnight!

My top ways to burst are:

- Run up the stairs.
- Sprint or run.
- Bike.
- Rollerblade like the Olympic speed skaters.
- Swim the butterfly stroke in the pool.
- Crank up the StairMaster.
- Jump rope.

## Resistance Training Gets Results

Putting on muscle mass is the most amazing thing that you can do for your metabolism. It holds everything in tighter, making you look firmer and leaner. And muscle requires more energy to exist on your body, so it raises your metabolic rate all day long. Resistance training can help improve insulin sensitivity, which aids with fat burning as well.

Sometimes I feel like I should put blinders on when I go to the gym because I see people doing the craziest things. Some are just plain ineffective and inefficient, and others are downright dangerous. I have created a basic video of the most common exercises and how to do them correctly that you can view at www.thevirgindiet.com/resistance.

I have divided the body into four functional groups: upper body pushing (chest, shoulders and triceps), upper body pulling (latissumus dorsi, upper back and biceps), hips and thighs and core/trunk.

Below are my core principles for getting the most from every workout. Just to clarify some of the common gym lingo, a set is when you repeat an exercise consistently for a certain amount of repetitions, or reps. For example, if I have you lift a weight once, that is 1 repetition. If I have you lift it twice, that is 2 repetitions. I might give you a set of 8 repetitions, ask you to recover for 60 seconds and then ask you to do another set of 8 reps. The principles below should help you design your own workouts, showing you how to get the most from each set, how to vary your sets and how to take breaks between your sets.

## JJ'S CORE PRINCIPLES FOR WORKING OUT

- Lift the heaviest weight you can safely handle in good form.

- Work between 8 and 12 repetitions per set. If you can't get to 8, lighten your load. If you get to 12 and feel like you could do another, add some additional weight.

If you are just starting, begin with 1 set of 8 to 12 reps of 2 to 3 exercises from each functional group for the first week and then increase to 2 sets.

- You can split your workouts up so you do two functional groups one day and two functional groups the next. It should feel easy to medium to start. It is always better to start slow and see how your body feels the next day. Progress to 2 sets and then begin increasing the resistance (the amount of weight lifted).

- Focus on free-weight and cable-style exercises rather than machines.

- Create a progressively more unstable environment. Basically, you want to have to work harder and harder to have to keep your balance, which means that you will be using more of your core muscles. (Your core muscles are your abdominal muscles and the muscles in your lower back.) For example, you can start by sitting, which requires the least effort from you to stay balanced. Then, do the same exercise standing up. Now you have to work a bit harder to keep standing while you complete the exercise. Next, you could sit on a big exercise ball. The ball will roll around a little, and you'll have to work hard to keep it stable as you exercise—and that work will involve your core muscles, which is great! Finally, try the same exercise standing on a BOSU ball, which is a ball cut in half with a flat side that rests on the floor and a round side that you stand on. Standing on a BOSU ball means that your core muscles will be working even harder, which will increase the value of your workout, build more muscle, boost your metabolism and greatly speed your weight loss.

- Give yourself 60 seconds to recover in between sets. You don't want to allow your muscles to fully recover between sets, you want to keep them working hard throughout the whole exercise session. But you do need short breaks so you can push yourself as hard as possible when you are doing the sets.

- If you're brand new to exercise, start with 1 set the first week, but after that always do multiple sets. That way, you will recruit more muscle fibers for better hypertrophy (muscle mass development). If you do just a single set, you don't involve as much of the muscle as when you repeat a set.

- Change things ups. Don't let your workout become routine:
  - Add new exercises at least every month.

- Superset: Alternate between two exercises of opposing muscle groups. For example, you might alternate between push-ups and pull-ups.
- Every few weeks, rotate in an endurance day, when you are working with less intensity but for a longer time. For example, lighten your load by 10 to 20 percent, but instead of doing 8 to 12 reps, do 2 sets of 15 to 25 reps for each exercise.
- Every few weeks, rotate in a super-strength day. For example, increase your load by 10 to 20 percent and do 4 to 6 sets of 3 to 6 reps for each exercise.
- Add some power exercises, such as burpees, medicine ball throws, kettle bell, squat thrusts and Turkish get-ups (see www.thevirgindiet.com/resistance for instructions).

• Your workout should never get easier. You can continue to up the intensity by progressing into a more unstable environment where you have to work harder to keep your balance, by increasing the weight and by adding in some power/plyometric training.

• Hit each functional group of muscles (the four groups I identified earlier) at least 2 times per week and ideally 3 times per week with 48 hours of rest in between.

• If you feel yourself stagnating or just have trouble getting started, hire a trainer to check your form and uplevel your workout. This is a great way to learn new exercises and get a push.

• Listen to your body. If you are sore to the touch or at a joint site, you have overdone it and need to back off and rest to recover. Try soaking in 1 or 2 cups of Epsom salts and warm water for 20 to 30 minutes.

## DON'T TELL ME YOU DON'T HAVE TIME!

If you absolutely don't have time to exercise, guess what? You still do! You can click on www.thevirgindiet.com/4x4 and get my free 4x4 Workout, which takes at most 15 minutes—even including some stretching—and which you only have to do 3 times per week. You can do it at home, so no travel time to the gym or park, and it requires very little equipment.

I call this workout "fast, fun and done in 15 minutes or less," although I will admit the fun is somewhat debatable. It includes burst training that uses your hips and thighs, resistance training for the four functional groups and a bit of stretching. You have time for this. If not, then make time. I won't take no for an answer, and now you have *no* excuses! You can thank me later.

## CHANGE IT UP!

Once you've got a good workout plan going, you need to change it up a little bit every 3 months or so. It is easy to get into a workout rut, but you need to continuously challenge yourself. Otherwise, your body gets used to what you're doing, and you don't get the same impact.

There are all kinds of fun ways to create new workouts. Consider cross-fit training or kettle bell workouts. Download workout ideas from online, take a new fitness class or hire a trainer. The best use of a trainer is to have him or her give you a new workout either once a week or once a month. They can kick your butt and show you some new exercises.

I travel all the time, and I use that as an opportunity to mix up my workouts. I try to take advantage of a great new place to hike, some unexpected place I can rollerblade or a gym that I've never been to before. You can find your own way of changing things up that fits into your life.

The one thing that you shouldn't do is get stuck in a rut. If you continue to do the same things, you will continue to get the same results. I look at aging as a big snowball going downhill. If you want to fight the momentum, you have to build some countermomentum—and you can't do that by sticking with the same thing.

## KEEPING THE VIRGIN DIET FUN

Diets are like dating, but maintenance is like marriage. Each cycle requires different habits because the behaviors that got you thin are not the same as the behaviors that keep you thin. And the rewards of dieting—watching the numbers on that scale go down or buying yourself a bunch of new outfits—are not the same as the rewards of maintenance. So, make sure you find ways to stay committed to your new habits, including the rewards we talked about in the last chapter.

Here's the most important habit to maintain: your weekly weigh-in. This is one that I personally had to learn the hard way. I used to own a gym, and for some reason, I thought that exempted me from my weekly appointment with a scale. To show my customers the results that they could expect, I wore spandex every day. Then, after a couple of scale-free months, I had to put on my jeans. Oops! I thought, *Did these just come out of the dryer?* Well, guess what? Every pair of jeans I owned felt like they had just come out of the dryer because I had unknowingly gained weight. So now, every week, I get on that scale.

What if you're running out of steam and still have some weight to lose? You can throw in some fun plateau busters:

- Replace 2 meals per day with Virgin Diet Shakes.
- Double up your workouts: do some bursting in the morning and resistance training in the afternoon.
- Increase the intensity of your workouts.
- Replace your high-fiber starchy carbs with more nonstarchy veggies.
- Drink more green tea to help boost your metabolism. I love it iced!
- Try my metabolic booster supplement bundle (see the Resources section on my website).
- Up your fiber.
- Make sure to drink half of your weight or more in water each day.
- Lighten up a bit by shifting from higher fat animal protein, such as grass-fed beef and lamb, to lower fat chicken breasts, turkey breasts and scallops.

You can also do a challenge with some friends if you want to get to the next level. Support each other and then celebrate together when the plateau is busted.

 ## SUSTAINING YOUR SUCCESS

Now we're almost at the end of our journey, but I don't really want the journey to end—not for you or for us together. So let me end this chapter with two invitations. First, I am always there for you on my website at www.thevirgindiet.com, with lots of information, motivation, help and support.

Second, whether you keep going with me or without me, *I want you to keep going*. We call Cycle 3 the Virgin Diet for Life cycle, but maybe we should call it the "lifetime forward movement cycle" because in my experience, you're either moving forward or moving backward. I don't want you to be moving backward. That means you need to keep moving forward.

Do you want to know one of my favorite statements ever? "Weight loss is a metaphor for life." I love this! One thing I've learned in my life is that how you do one thing is how you do everything. If you commit to yourself to lose weight, look younger and feel terrific, it won't just be your health that benefits—it will be your whole life. Many of my clients have found that their whole lives changed. I've seen it over and over again: as you start to put yourself at the top of the list, things shift.

I've seen this kind of powerful transformation all the time in my clients. It's the kind of change that I want to see for you.

**You can be better now than you've ever been in your life.**

I want you to get inspired to stick with this for life, so here is my shot at inspiring you: I believe you can be better now than you've ever been in your life. We are so much smarter. We have great science now to back us up. I know I look better now than I did in high school, in college, in my 20s or in my 30s. I'm almost 50, and I think it's been a journey of continual improvement. Yes, I faced some bumps along the road, but in the end, all my setbacks made me stronger. The same can be true for you. So please, don't limit yourself. Don't believe it when people say, "You're gaining weight. That's the way it is. You will always look that way. That's aging." Don't accept that because it's simply not true.

At the same time, you need to be prepared for some bumps along the road because they eventually happen to everybody in some form or other, and I don't want you to be discouraged by them. You might be under stress. You may go through andropause or menopause. You can go through those difficult times and come out stronger and better than when you went in. The important thing is to figure out your own definition of personal best and not let anyone else impose their limitations on you.

Making this kind of change will change everything. When you are your best self emotionally, physically and spiritually, you can achieve your life's purpose. There is nothing more important.

Whether our purpose is giving to charity, doing some type of work or raising kids, there are messages that we are supposed to pass on to the world in some way. If you're not fulfilling your purpose, you're denying your best self—and that's never a good thing to do.

In his book *Lead the Field,* inspirational author and speaker Earl Nightingale says that we're never better than when we're facing a challenge. After we achieve our goal, we're a bit depressed, so we need to go on to set the next one. Well, now you've created this amazing achievement for yourself: you've finished the first three cycles of the Virgin Diet. That's awesome! I'm proud of you. So now, what's your next challenge? I want you to say to yourself, *If I could do that, what can I do now? Can I ramp up my exercise to the next level? Do I share my newfound love of health with others?*

Make sure that you are the person who makes other people say, "I want to have what she's having!" Make sure that you are making better choices, taking care of your body, putting yourself first, getting enough sleep and having balance in your life that is not all work and no play. So, what is your new identity? Now it's up to you!

# THE VIRGIN DIET MEAL ASSEMBLIES
## AND RESTAURANT GUIDE

## 11

Now it's time to put it all together! I don't want you to stress out in the kitchen, so I'm focusing on quick and easy-to-fix choices. In the following pages, you will find some sample meal assemblies. As you can see, each one is based on assembling items from a number of categories: clean, lean proteins; high-fiber, low-glycemic carbs; healthy fats; and nonstarchy vegetables. You can assemble any of these choices for any meal. Just remember that you are also including one or two Virgin Diet Shakes in your daily diet and don't forget to follow the Golden Rules of Meal Timing.

I've also included some of my favorite recipes in Chapter 12. And to make grocery shopping easier, turn to page 293 for The Virgin Diet Shopping List.

# THE ULTIMATE MEAL ASSEMBLY GUIDE

## ASSEMBLY BASICS

### CLEAN, LEAN PROTEIN
4-6 ounces for women
6-8 ounces for men
(go for the higher end of the range if you are very
athletic with higher muscle mass or if you are
50 or more pounds overweight)

**+**

### HIGH-FIBER, LOW-GLYCEMIC CARBS
½ cup for women
1 cup for men

**+**

### 1-3 SERVINGS OF HEALTHY FAT
1 serving = 100 calories
(1 serving = 1 tablespoon of fat = ⅓ avocado;
the fat contained in grass-fed beef, pasture-fed pork,
lamb or wild cold-water fish counts as 1 serving)

**+**

### NONSTARCHY VEGETABLES
2+ cups raw OR

1+ cups cooked
(the more the better here as I would like to see you have
at least 5 and ideally 10 servings per day...so load up!)

Assemble your meals from clean, lean protein; high-fiber, low-glycemic carbs; healthy fats; and nonstarchy vegetables. Here is a list of some acceptable choices that you can use in meal assembly, followed by some suggestions for how to put your meals together:

## CLEAN, LEAN PROTEIN

| | |
|---|---|
| Chicken breast | Roast beef slices |
| Grass-fed beef tenderloin | Sole |
| King crab | Turkey slices |
| Pasture-fed pork loin | Wild salmon |
| Pea-rice protein powder | Wild scallops |

## HIGH-FIBER, LOW-GLYCEMIC CARBS

| | |
|---|---|
| Apples and other moderate GI fruit | Kabocha squash |
| Beets | Lentils |
| Berries | Quinoa |
| Black beans | Quinoa pasta |
| Brown rice | Rice noodles |
| Butternut squash | Sweet potato |
| Hummus | Tomatoes |

## HEALTHY FATS

| | |
|---|---|
| Avocado | Grass-fed beef |
| Coconut milk | Nut butter |
| Coconut oil | Nuts |
| Cold-water fish | Palm fruit oil |
| Extra-virgin olive oil | Seeds |

## NONSTARCHY VEGETABLES

| | |
|---|---|
| Arugula | Red onions |
| Asparagus | Red peppers |
| Broccoli | Roasted cauliflower |
| Broccolini | Romaine |
| Brussels sprouts | Sautéed green beans, mushrooms |
| Chopped veggies | and garlic |
| Cripsy kale chips | Sautéed kale |
| Grilled veggie medley | Sautéed red, rainbow or Swiss chard |
| Mixed greens | Sautéed spinach and garlic |
| Mushrooms | Summer squash |

## THE BOWL

### CHOOSE BROWN RICE, QUINOA OR LEGUMES AS BASE

| + | Add stir-fried, steamed, roasted or sautéed vegetables. |
|---|---|
| + | Add your protein. |
| + | Add your healthy fat. |
| + | Top with your sauce or seasoning. |

I've made it super simple to restock your kitchen with the staples you need to succeed on the Virgin Diet. You can download my list at www.thevirgindiet.com/shoppinglist and take it with you to the grocery store.

### MY FAVORITE BOWL

- Quinoa (steam in chicken or veggie broth)
- Roasted Brussels sprouts, asparagus, red peppers (roast in palm fruit or coconut oil)
- Grilled salmon
- Lemon and sea salt

## SAUCES AND SEASONINGS

Great spices and seasoning blends can make you forget all about the 7 high-FI foods. The challenge is that spice blends can also be a source of hidden gluten, sugar, soy and dairy, so you must make sure you read the labels carefully.

I know I'm asking you to eat in a whole new way, and I'd like to make your decisions as simple as possible. I'd also like to retool your palate to appreciate the fresh and subtle flavors of clean, lean proteins; high-fiber, low-glycemic carbs; healthy fats; and nonstarchy veggies. So for Cycles 1 and 2 of the zero tolerance diet, you will ideally make your own sauces and seasonings using your favorite vinegars, extra-virgin olive oil, fresh lemon and lime juice, coconut milk and spices. Not only will you save money by not buying a lot of canned and bottled sauces, but you will also unleash your creativity and know exactly what you are getting!

It's harder than you might think to find prepared sauces and seasonings that don't contain hidden traps. A lot of spice blends contain MSG, which is a highly reactive food for many people. Many sauces contain gluten, egg, dairy, peanuts or soy, which are sometimes listed on the label but sometimes hidden (rules vary about what kinds of ingredients have to be listed). So for these first two phases, stick to the specific sauce that I've recommended in the shopping list on page 294 and to single-ingredient spices rather than blends—ideally, nonirradiated and organic. You can make an exception for salsas, marinara sauce and guacamole, which are usually fine, but watch for corn in the salsa, and sugar and cheese in the marinara. By the way, ketchups are always made with sugar, so use marinara or salsa instead.

In Cycle 3, you can experiment a bit more freely with some prepared sauces. In Cycles 1 and 2, however, go lean to go clean! You're in for a whole new world of taste—enjoy!

# THE PLATE

PROTEIN

| + | Allowable high-fiber, starchy carbohydrate choices |
|---|---|
| + | Veggies |
| + | Healthy fat, such as olive oil, avocado or nuts |

## MY FAVORITE PLATE

- Grass-fed beef fillet
- ½ sweet potato
- Asparagus, lightly sautéed with olive oil
- Garlic and sea salt

## THE SALAD

START WITH DEEP GREEN LEAFIES

| + | Add chopped or julienned nonstarchy veggies. |
|---|---|
| + | Throw in a little high-fiber carb. |
| + | Add protein. |
| + | Add healthy fat (nuts, avocado and/or dressing). |
| + | Dress and season. |

### MY FAVORITE SALAD

- Romaine and spinach blend
- Chopped cucumbers, red onions, red peppers, carrots and some asparagus, steamed al dente and chilled
- Garbanzo beans
- Diced chicken
- Sliced avocado
- Lemon, olive oil and basil to dress

## STEER CLEAR OF ICEBERG

Iceberg lettuce has close to zero nutritional value and is pretty much just a delivery system for pesticides. Plus, why would you choose iceberg when there are so many more delicious and nutritious lettuces? My favorites include peppery arugula, potassium-rich radicchio, spinach greens, kale and my favorite standby, hearts of romaine.

## THE STOUP: PART STEW, PART SOUP

CHICKEN OR VEGGIE BROTH

| + | Add lentils, legumes, brown rice or quinoa. |
|---|---|
| + | Add nonstarchy veggies (load up!). |
| + | Add chopped protein. |
| + | Serve with a side salad with extra-virgin olive oil, lemon juice and a tablespoon of chopped walnuts. |

## MY FAVORITE STOUP

- Low-sodium, organic chicken broth
- Lentils
- Sautéed, chopped onions, garlic, red and yellow peppers and zucchini
- Diced, roasted chicken breast
- Side salad (mixed field greens and herb salad with 1 tablespoon chopped walnuts)

# THE WRAP

START WITH RICE WRAP, ROMAINE OR BUTTER LEAF LETTUCE

| + | Add protein. |
| --- | --- |
| + | Add chopped nonstarchy veggies and leafy greens. |
| + | Add healthy fat, such as chopped nuts or avocado. |

## MY FAVORITE WRAP

- Rice wrap
- Turkey slices
- Arugula, basil and heirloom tomato
- Sliced avocado
- Gluten-free Dijon mustard

# SNACKS

Think of these as a minimeal. Your snacks should include: 0 or 1 starchy carb, 2 to 4 ounces protein, 1 fat and lots of nonstarchy veggies.

## SOME SNACK IDEAS:

- Celery with hummus
- Apples with almond butter
- Minishake (one-half of the normal recipe)
- Cup of lentil soup (See the Resources section on my website for some gluten-free brands.)
- Turkey rollup (a slice of turkey rolled up with a slice of avocado and a slice of tomato)
- Freeze-dried berries mixed with raw nuts
- Crudités with black bean dip or guacamole

# COOL SUBSTITUTIONS

Don't worry, you don't have to give up all of your faves to achieve your ideal weight and maintain it for life. Part of the success of this program is training yourself to think about food and what's really healthy in a new way, and there are lots of healthy substitutions that will leave you feeling satisfied and slim at the same time. Here are some of my favorite ways of subbing in a healing or low-FI choice instead of a high-FI one. So, swap and enjoy!

## INSTEAD OF MILK OR SOY MILK...

I am not a fan of rice, hemp or most almond milks. They often contain too much sugar, and even the sugar-free ones are carb dumps. I don't see the nutritional benefit. Drink coconut milk instead. Coconut milk is a rock star—just make sure that it's unsweetened.

## INSTEAD OF MASHED POTATOES...

Milky, creamy mashed potatoes are high-glycemic. Would you eat ice cream as a side dish for dinner? Well, the sugar in the potato plus the added pro-inflammatory fat to mash them makes this food choice way too unhealthy for anything but an occasional dessert. Trade your mashed potatoes and milk for mashed cauliflower with olive oil or coconut milk.

## INSTEAD OF POTATO CHIPS...

This favorite salty treat is made out of potatoes, and as far as I'm concerned, a potato is just a big lump of sugar. Do you know what sugar does inside your body? It turns almost immediately into fat. So I say, pass on the potato chips. Instead, roast some finely chopped Brussels sprouts until they are crunchy to satisfy your chip craving. I have turned the most die-hard Brussels sprouts haters into fans with these (and saved the most die-hard chip addicts with them, too!). Roasted kale seasoned with sea salt is another nutrient-dense chip alternative. (See the recipe on page 271.)

## INSTEAD OF PIES...

If you love pie, you can bake apples, peaches, blueberries, sweet potatoes or a mix of these to satisfy your sweet craving. Try using cinnamon instead of sugar or perhaps add a dash of unsweetened vanilla extract. Nutmeg and cloves also give the fruit a little extra zing. Then, use crunchy nuts on the top or bottom as a crust. It is delicious, like a graham cracker crust. Or you can make your own crust with almond flour, coconut oil and vanilla. (See the recipe on page 282.)

Here are a few more cool substitutions:

- Instead of soy sauce, try coconut aminos (see the Resources section on my website).
- Instead of cow's or goat's milk yogurt, have coconut yogurt.
- Instead of flours with gluten, have almond or coconut flour.
- Instead of peanut butter, have almond butter, cashew butter or macadamia nut butter.
- Instead of regular butter, try ghee (clarified butter), hummus or guacamole.
- Instead of ketchup, try marinara or salsa.
- Instead of pasta, try spaghetti squash.
- If you like sandwiches, wraps or pitas, try lettuce wraps.
- For little pizzas, use sliced eggplant, portobello mushrooms or a rice cake.

- If you love hot chocolate, you will adore vegan pea–rice chocolate powder with coconut milk. It is amazing.
- If you're addicted to frappuccinos or coffee mocha drinks, try coffee powder mixed with coconut milk, cinnamon, chocolate protein powder and ice. You can either do it shaken or blended. Either way, it is awesome.

 ## THE SKINNY ON DRINKS

Okay, you're committing yourself to 64 ounces of water each day—either plain or the sparkling kind in the glass bottles. (See Doing Water Right on pages 173–174.) Now, what else can you drink?

You don't have to cut caffeine out altogether (I certainly haven't) because it's actually good for weight loss—*in low doses*. So, I want you to get down to a reasonable amount—about one or two cups of coffee or green tea per day. Again, take it slow. Start by switching to half caffeine/half decaf. If you have tea or coffee in the afternoon, transition to decaf or caffeine-free and only drink the strong stuff in the morning.

Cutting back on the caffeine is important for weight loss because higher levels of caffeine can raise your stress hormones and keep them up, which can lead to higher fasting blood sugar levels and weight gain. Caffeine can also disrupt sleep, which also raises stress hormones. So, all the good you are doing with your Virgin Diet and your healing foods could be undone by too much caffeine.

- **Green tea.** I love green tea! The studies are amazing on green tea. It helps improve insulin sensitivity, it helps your body handle stress better, it is a great antioxidant, and it lowers appetite and boosts metabolism.

- **Coffee.** I fight with my fellow nutritionists often about this. I believe that coffee is a health food—in the right amounts. It is a very rich antioxidant crop. But the right amounts are crucial: 1 or 2 cups is great, 5 cups is a problem, and a whole pot of coffee is a big problem.

  Buy organic coffee. Coffee beans are a very pesticide-laden crop.

  I personally get Americanos because espresso is lower in caffeine. My own preference is a half-decaf Americano, or if I want a treat in the afternoon, I have an iced decaf Americano.

  So, you can have your coffee as long as you watch the dose and don't turn it into dessert by loading it with syrups, milk and sugar. A little xylitol, stevia and coconut milk are fine. Track your coffee intake, your mood and your sleep habits in your food journal. If you're feeling jumpy or not sleeping well, switch to decaf.

- **Alcohol.** In Cycles 1 and 2, I want you to pass on the alcohol. A healthy liver is essential for metabolizing fat and processing toxins, which will help speed your weight loss, so for the next 3 weeks, I want you to give your liver a rest. Plus, I've often found that drinking can cloud your judgment and make it easier to indulge. Check out pages 215–216 in Chapter 10 for the good news about what you *can* drink in Cycle 3!

- **Green drinks.** I love these. I want people to have 10 servings of nonstarchy vegetables per day, and green drinks are a great way to boost your intake. They are also very detoxifying. You want to be careful to have a green drink that's all green. I find that most green drinks are just juice in disguise. A green drink should contain cabbage, kale, broccoli, spinach and celery. No beets, apples, carrots or any of the other high-glycemic vegetables or fruits. Find a juice bar to get fresh green drinks or make them at home if you have a juicer. You can even do the powdered green drinks as long as they don't have sugar in them.

If you are juicing at home, toss in some fresh ginger to help soothe and heal your gastrointestinal tract. Plus, it adds a great little zing! If you are really adventurous and don't have a hot date, add some fresh garlic as well.

## JJ'S TIPS FOR DINING OUT

I'm on the road all the time, and more of my meals are eaten out than in. So, I don't want to hear any excuses about a restaurant lifestyle keeping you from following the Virgin Diet! If I can do it, so can you—and I'm going to help you.

This doesn't mean that you can throw caution to the wind and order a double cheeseburger, fries and then that monster piece of cheese-cake for dessert. There are easy ways to dine at restaurants and eat healthy and wonderful creations while you continue to follow the plan and enjoy the company of your family and friends (and avoid doing the dishes!).

Here are my favorite tips for eating out:

- **Survey the entire menu when you sit down.** You don't have to stick to whatever side dish is listed with a specific entrée. Let's say you want the salmon, which comes with high-FI risotto, but the steak dinner has a great side of sautéed spinach and garlic. You can easily ask your server to switch the sides.

- **Always start with a salad with olive oil and lemon juice or your favorite vinegar.** Beware of salad killers that up the calories, including sugared nuts, bacon, tortilla strips, rice noodles and wontons. Pass on the creamy salad dressings and be careful of sugary vinaigrettes (raspberry, Asian and so on). Order olive oil and vinegar and/or lemon on the side and make your own dressing.

- **Double your veggies and skip the starch.** Ask for 2 servings of veggies as your side instead of the starch. You really don't need the loaded potato or the buttery rice.

- **Try a new veggie that you don't normally make in your kitchen.** If kale is a question mark, then try it when you're out. Make this an adventure.

- **Never order anything with these words attached to them:** *breaded, fried, crunchy, crispy, glazed* or *creamy.* That saves you a world of trouble right there.

- **Never assume.** Before I learned this one, I was unpleasantly surprised all too often. I'd order "simply broiled" fish and discover that it was loaded with butter. I'd ask for a dish described as "chicken breast sautéed in olive oil" and find out that it had been dipped in egg and breadcrumbs before it went into the oil. I've found unannounced croutons in my salad and unexpected crème fraîche garnishing my soup. Explain your dietary needs to the server and then repeat the same questions for every single dish: Does it have dairy? Does it have eggs? Is there any wheat or bread in there? Does it have soy? Remember, ignorance is never an excuse!

- **Don't invite the enemy to the table.** Send the bread basket away before it even touches the table. Don't even invite the temptation.

- **Pick two appetizers as your main course for better portion control.** Choose wisely to make sure you get some high-quality proteins and some healthy veggies. For example, you might ask for hummus with veggies and grilled chicken kabobs with salsa.

- **Share a large entrée with a friend who has a very fast fork.** Let your friend have the last bite. Your waistline will thank you for it.

- **Take home half of your protein portion and extra veggies.** Use them to make a yummy wrap for lunch the next day. I love to take grilled chicken and veggies home and put them into a brown rice wrap.

Sound good? I hope so! Check, please!

If you want specific suggestions for specific types of restaurants, check out www.thevirgindiet.com/diningout.

 ## "BUT I DON'T WANT TO SEEM DIFFICULT…": HANDLING THOSE TRICKY SITUATIONS

You've been invited to your cousin's wedding, and you're not about to ask her for a special meal. You're eating at your boyfriend's mom's house, and you don't want to look like a picky eater. You're joining a group of coworkers for lunch at your new job, and they've chosen a restaurant with a menu that seems to be totally off-limits. Now what?

Believe me, I've been there! Many, many times.

There will always be food pushers. Sometimes they even love you. Sometimes people who would never think of pushing you to have a cigarette or take a drink or do something dangerous will try to push food on you, saying, "A little bit can't hurt."

I've found that if you don't make a big deal out of it, no one else will either. When you frame your response in terms of health rather than weight, it lets you off the hook. If you say you're on a diet or trying to lose 5 pounds, people will try to spoon-feed you cake. Instead, tell them the truth. Say something like, "I've been having a lot of pain, inflammation and gastrointestinal problems. It looks like it's linked to some of the foods that I've been eating. My body doesn't tolerate them well. Right now I can't touch them while I'm going through this healing phase. If I do, it will mess up the whole process and hurt me." Or if you're not comfortable disclosing so many details, you can say, "I love that you're concerned, but you know, this is a tough topic for me. Would it be okay if we didn't talk about it?"

Sometimes you don't have to say anything—just avoid the high-FI foods. If I'm going to a sit-down dinner, I explain it to the hostess ahead of time. If I show up at someone's home and they offer me some food I can't eat, I might just say, "No, thank you," or I might quietly explain that I have a health issue so they won't wonder why I am refusing all of their food.

What about those times when you're joining some people at a restaurant and you can't find anything on the menu that fits your plan? Be creative. Charm the server into arranging a plain piece of meat, chicken or fish with no sauce and no butter, plus a plain salad with a lemon

> If you're clear about your purpose and your intention, you can handle any obstacle.

wedge and maybe some olive oil. It might not be the best restaurant meal in the world, but you're there to enjoy the company more. And you might be surprised—there are usually some absolutely fabulous choices.

If you're clear about your purpose and your intention, you can handle any obstacle that gets thrown in your path.

There are also food pushers and saboteurs out there who don't care about you losing weight and feeling better, who may even prefer you stay heavy and unhealthy. Don't let them define your choices. You define your own choices. You'll look better *and* feel better if you do.

## LOOKING FORWARD TO A NEW YOU

Every person I've ever pulled off the 7 high-FI foods gets better in some way. Every single person. So trust me, you will feel better.

You'll feel even better if you track your symptoms right from the start. If you haven't already done so, take the quiz in Chapter 1 and notice what you're tolerating. You're going to notice the weight loss, I promise you. But what about the other incredible benefits from this diet? They're

> Trust me, you will feel better.

usually shocking to people. They didn't realize that these things could be fixed. They figured these problems were normal for them.

If you need another reminder of how to get yourself started, go back to Chapter 2 and get your support system in place. Find an accountability buddy and join my support forum at www.thevirgindiet.com/forum. Set up your food journal and your tracking system. (Grab these at www.thevirgindiet.com/journal and www.thevirgindiet.com/weighttracker.) Throw all the wrong foods out of your kitchen and pantry and prepare to make a fresh start.

A wonderful healing journey is about to begin. In 21 days, you'll be 10 to 15 pounds lighter, look 10 years younger and feel better than you've felt in a long, long time.

# HOW THE VIRGIN DIET WORKED FOR ME

Valene Middleton
Age 33

Springville,
Washington

**Height:**
5'5"

**Starting Weight:**
143 pounds

**Waist:** 35"
**Hips:** 37"

**Current Weight:**
124 pounds

**Waist:** 31.5"
**Hips:** 34.5"

**Lost:** 19 pounds

I am so grateful for JJ's diet plan! I tried going off gluten, dairy, citrus and nuts a few years ago and it was a miserable experience. I had no idea what to eat. The products I bought from the then hard-to-find gluten-free sections of the store were all nasty. Everything was very expensive, and I felt totally lost. And it didn't even help!

This experience has been very different than my last attempt. The food has been so great that when a colleague invited my husband and me to go out to dinner, my husband replied that he didn't know if we could find restaurant food as good as what I have been making.

Thanks to JJ's approach, the bloating is gone and my gastrointestinal issues are a whole lot better.

Before starting the Virgin Diet, I saw disease specialists, family practioners, a gastrointestinal specialist, a nutritionist and a holistic chiropractor, and none of them were able to help me.

I started the Virgin Diet hoping to reduce my major symptoms and it's worked. I didn't really expect any weight loss, but it happened anyway! At 19 pounds lighter, my pants are now falling off!

My husband has eaten more vegetables since I started the program than he has in his entire life. We have both eaten veggies that we had never tried before. It's been good for the whole family.

JJ and her program did what all those doctors and specialists could not. She provided me with the information and support I needed to feel better and bring about the changes I wanted to make in my life. I will always be grateful for that.

# THE VIRGIN DIET RECIPES

## 12

If you are in the mood to cook, I have included some of my favorite creations that are still simple but a step up from my time-saving meal assembly. You will notice that my serving sizes are a bit bigger for the salads and veggies because I want you to eat 5 to 10 servings per day from the rainbow of nonstarchy veggies!

# RECIPES FOR CYCLE 1: ELIMINATION

## BREAKFAST

## THE VIRGIN DIET SHAKE

### INGREDIENTS

1 to 2 scoops vegan pea–rice protein powder*

1 to 2 tablespoons** fiber (fiber blend, chia seeds, hemp seeds, freshly ground flaxseed meal or nut butter)

$\frac{1}{2}$ to 1 cup organic frozen berries

1 cup liquid (water, unsweetened coconut milk*** or coconut water)

### OPTIONAL

Add 1 cup frozen chopped spinach or fresh kale—you won't even taste it!

### DIRECTIONS

Blend and drink.

### VARIATIONS

**If you like your shake thinner**

1 to 2 scoops protein

1 serving fiber

$\frac{1}{2}$ cup organic frozen fruit

10 ounces liquid

**If you like your shake thicker**

1 to 2 scoops protein

1 serving fiber

1 serving chia, hemp or freshly ground flaxseeds

1 cup organic frozen fruit

8 ounces liquid

Ice cubes

* Aim for 20-25 grams of protein per shake.
** I really want you to pump up your fiber so build up to those 2 tablespoons per shake.
*** I recommend So Delicious unsweetened coconut milk. If you use the canned coconut milk, choose the light version and dilute $\frac{1}{4}$ cup coconut milk to $\frac{3}{4}$ cup water.

## PROTEIN POWER OATMEAL

SERVES
(1)

### INGREDIENTS

Gluten-free oatmeal*

1 teaspoon cinnamon

1 to 2 tablespoons chopped nuts (almonds, pecans, walnuts)

1 scoop vanilla vegan protein powder, liquefied in $\frac{1}{4}$ cup water**

### DIRECTIONS

Prepare oatmeal as directed for 1 serving. Toward the end of cooking, add cinnamon.

Remove from heat and add chopped nuts and liquefied protein powder. Stir well.

Add more water if needed for desired consistency.

* Be sure to buy gluten-free long-cooking or steel-cut oats.
** You can substitute coconut milk for water.

## WARM SHAKE

SERVES
(1)

### INGREDIENTS

1 cup frozen berries (any type) and/or dark cherries

1 teaspoon cinnamon

$\frac{1}{2}$ cup coconut milk

1 scoop vanilla vegan protein powder

1 tablespoon chia seeds

1 tablespoon chopped walnuts

### DIRECTIONS

Warm cherries/berries and coconut milk over medium heat until fruit is warm.

Pour off a few tablespoons of liquid and combine with the vegan protein powder. Whisk until smooth and add back to mixture.

Stir in chia seeds, cinnamon and chopped walnuts.

# SALADS AND SALAD DRESSINGS

## EVERYDAY VINAIGRETTE

### INGREDIENTS

2 tablespoons + 1 teaspoon vinegar (balsamic, red wine, champagne, etc.)

$\frac{1}{2}$ cup extra-virgin olive oil

$\frac{1}{2}$ teaspoon sea salt

$\frac{1}{2}$ teaspoon freshly cracked black pepper

### DIRECTIONS

Whisk all ingredients together.

### VARIATIONS

**Vinaigrette Dijon**
Add 2 tablespoons grainy Dijon mustard.

**Garlic Basil Vinaigrette**
Add 1 minced garlic clove and 1 bunch chopped fresh basil.

**Country French Vinaigrette**
Add 1 teaspoon herbs de Provence.

## JJ'S BASIC SALAD

SERVES

### INGREDIENTS

4 cups romaine or mixed baby greens

2 tablespoons chopped walnuts or pecans

¼ sliced red onion

½ can hearts of palm or artichoke hearts

8 sliced radishes

If you are using as a main dish salad, add protein.

### DIRECTIONS

Toss all ingredients together with dressing on page 263 and serve.

## SUMMER KALE SALAD

SERVES

### INGREDIENTS

¼ cup lemon juice

1 teaspoon chopped, fresh oregano

¼ cup extra-virgin olive oil

1 teaspoon minced shallots

½ teaspoon stone-ground mustard

2 large bunches washed, chopped ¼" thick organic kale

¼ cup halved heirloom cherry tomatoes

½ cup finely chopped walnuts

Kale can be a bit bitter. If you like, you can blend with fresh spinach leaves.

### DIRECTIONS

In a small bowl, whisk together the lemon juice, oregano, olive oil, shallots and mustard until well combined.

To assemble the salad, lightly toss the kale with the vinaigrette.

Top with the heirloom tomatoes and walnuts.

## CHICORY LETTUCE SALAD

SERVES
2

### INGREDIENTS

3 cups frisée lettuce

1 cup chicory lettuce

¼ cup extra-virgin olive oil

1 tablespoon sherry vinegar

1 teaspoon minced shallots

### DIRECTIONS

Blend the lettuces in a large bowl.

In a small bowl, mix the olive oil, vinegar and shallots.

Lightly toss the salad with this mix.

## TRIPLE CABBAGE SLAW

SERVES (2)

### INGREDIENTS

1 cup shredded Napa cabbage

1 cup shredded green cabbage

1 cup shredded red cabbage

3 sliced green onions

1 teaspoon freshly grated ginger (or dry powdered)

1 teaspoon apple cider vinegar

1 teaspoon extra-virgin olive oil

1/2 teaspoon sesame oil

### DIRECTIONS

In a medium bowl, mix shredded cabbages, green onions, ginger, vinegar, olive oil and sesame oil.

If you can, chill covered in the fridge for about 30 minutes to let the flavors marry and then serve chilled.

## CLASSIC GREEK SALAD

SERVES (2)

### INGREDIENTS

2 cucumbers, sliced into rounds and then quartered

1 cup thinly shaved red onion

1 diced, large heirloom tomato

1 teaspoon extra-virgin olive oil

1 teaspoon apple cider or sherry vinegar

### DIRECTIONS

Mix together in a medium bowl and serve.

## ASIAN SUMMER SALAD

SERVES (2) OR MORE

### INGREDIENTS

1 pound peeled, deveined jumbo shrimp

1 head Bibb lettuce

1/2 large pink grapefruit, peeled, segmented and cut into pieces

1/2 cup Chinese peapods

1 sliced avocado

2 tablespoons sliced almonds

4 pieces celery, chopped

1/2 julienned red pepper

1/2 deskinned, deseeded, diced cucumber

### DIRECTIONS

Combine all, toss gently with Asian dressing and serve immediately.

## GREEK-STYLE CHOPPED SALAD

SERVES
(2)

### INGREDIENTS

1 small head romaine, cut into ½" pieces

1 peeled, seeded cucumber, cut into ½" pieces

½ red bell pepper, cut into ½" pieces

½ yellow bell pepper, cut into ½" pieces

½ red onion, cut into ½" pieces

¼ cup chopped black olives

1½ tablespoons red wine vinegar

1 tablespoon extra-virgin olive oil

### DIRECTIONS

Combine all ingredients and toss gently.

# DIPS AND SNACKS

## BASIC HUMMUS DIP

SERVES
(4)

### INGREDIENTS

2 cups canned, drained garbanzo beans

⅓ cup tahini

¼ cup lemon juice

2 crushed cloves garlic

2 tablespoons extra-virgin olive oil

1 teaspoon sea salt

1 pinch paprika

### DIRECTIONS

Place the garbanzo beans, tahini, lemon juice, garlic, olive oil and sea salt in a blender or food processor.

Blend until smooth. Transfer mixture to a serving bowl and sprinkle with paprika.

Serve with cucumber, red pepper and jicama spears.

## ROASTED NUTS

### DIRECTIONS

Serving size can be adjusted based on amount of nuts.

Soak nuts of your choice overnight in water with sea salt and then drain the water.

Toss nuts in cinnamon (or pumpkin pie spice) and unsweetened vanilla extract or make them spicy and salty with curry powder and a little sea salt.

Spread onto a cookie sheet.

Bake at 140°F for 8 hours. Let cool and then store in the fridge.

# SOUPS

## FISH STEW WITH
### COCONUT MILK AND CILANTRO

SERVES
(4)

### INGREDIENTS

2 pounds fish (Salmon, scallops and shrimp are my favorite.)

4 tablespoons palm fruit or coconut oil, divided

1 large jar diced tomatoes (add fresh if available)

1 diced green pepper

1 diced red pepper

1 diced onion

2 crushed garlic cloves

1 can light coconut milk

1 cup unsweetened coconut milk (So Delicious or Trader Joe's)

1 teaspoon sea salt

### DIRECTIONS

Cook fish in 2 tablespoons oil for 2 ½ minutes per side at medium heat.

Next, sauté rest of oil, vegetables and garlic.

Add remaining ingredients and simmer on low heat for 30 minutes.

Add additional coconut milk if you would like it thinner.

Add red curry or red pepper flakes if you want a little zing.

## LENTIL SOUP

SERVES (4)

### INGREDIENTS

1 pound steamed lentils*

1 pound cooked, diced chicken breast

2 cups organic chicken broth

2 minced cloves garlic

2 tablespoons organic olive oil

½ cup chopped celery

½ cup diced onion

½ to 1 teaspoon sea salt

### DIRECTIONS

Combine lentils, chicken breast and chicken broth and start simmering.

Sauté garlic in olive oil until just golden.

Add celery and onion and cook until soft.

Add sea salt.

Add entire mixture to soup and simmer for 20 minutes.

* Trader Joe's sells these in the refrigerator section.

# VEGGIE SIDE DISHES

## RATATOUILLE

SERVES (4)

### INGREDIENTS

5 medium-diced plum tomatoes

1 medium-diced, large eggplant

2 medium-diced, large red onions

2 seeded, medium-diced red bell peppers

2 seeded, medium-diced yellow bell peppers

½ cup extra-virgin olive oil

6 sliced cloves garlic

1 teaspoon rosemary

1 teaspoon thyme

1 teaspoon basil

1 teaspoon sea salt

½ teaspoon freshly cracked black pepper

### DIRECTIONS

Combine all ingredients in casserole dish and bake at 350°F for 30 minutes.

## BRAISED RAINBOW CHARD

SERVES
(4)

### INGREDIENTS

3 minced cloves garlic

1 teaspoon olive oil

2 heads rainbow chard, chopped into 1" pieces

1 cup organic chicken stock

### DIRECTIONS

In a large pan on medium heat, gently sweat the garlic in the olive oil.

Add in the chard and stir so you help the leaves wilt.

Add in the chicken stock and cook for 10 minutes or until the liquid is mostly dissolved.

Season with sea salt and pepper if desired.

## ROASTED VEGETABLES

SERVES
(2)
OR MORE

### INGREDIENTS

2 cups 2 or more different veggies, cut into bite-sized chunks or julienned: Brussels sprouts (halved), cauliflower, zucchini, summer squash, asparagus, portobello mushrooms, red bell peppers, Japanese eggplant, onions

3 to 4 tablespoons coconut oil or Malaysian palm fruit oil

Sea salt to taste

### DIRECTIONS

Combine ingredients and spread out on a baking dish or two.

Bake at 400°F. Stir/turn at 30 minutes and continue to roast until desired doneness (depends on size of chunks).

## SAUTÉED SPINACH AND GARLIC

SERVES
(2)

### INGREDIENTS

2 tablespoons palm fruit oil

3 peeled, very thinly sliced cloves garlic

1¼ pounds spinach, stems trimmed off, well washed, dried

Generous pinch red pepper flakes

1 teaspoon sea salt

Freshly cracked black pepper to taste

### DIRECTIONS

Heat the palm fruit oil and garlic over high heat until very hot, almost smoking.

Add the spinach and cook, stirring rapidly, for about 1 to 2 minutes until the spinach turns bright green and wilts slightly.

Remove the spinach from the heat.

Add salt, pepper and red pepper flakes, and toss well to combine.

Serve immediately.

## SAUTÉED GREEN BEANS
### WITH MUSHROOMS AND GARLIC

SERVES
2

| INGREDIENTS | DIRECTIONS |
|---|---|
| 1 pound fresh green beans | Lightly steam green beans until al dente. |
| 4 peeled, thinly sliced cloves garlic | While green beans are steaming, sauté garlic in oil until light golden, add mushrooms and continue to sauté. |
| 1 to 2 tablespoons palm fruit or olive oil | |
| 1 pound sliced mushrooms (any type) | When mushrooms are tender, add drained green beans, salt and pepper and mix together. |
| 1 teaspoon sea salt | |
| ½ teaspoon freshly cracked black pepper | |

## SAUTÉED MUSHROOMS

 OR

SERVES
2
SIDES

SERVES
4
TOPPINGS

| INGREDIENTS | DIRECTIONS |
|---|---|
| 1 tablespoon olive or palm fruit oil | Heat oil in large skillet over medium heat. |
| 2 minced cloves garlic | Add garlic and cook 1 minute. |
| 2 cups mixed wild mushrooms | Add mushrooms and cook 3 to 5 minutes, until tender. |
| 1 tablespoon dry sherry or organic chicken broth | Add sherry or chicken broth about halfway through. |
| 1 teaspoon sea salt | Season with salt and black pepper. |
| ½ teaspoon freshly cracked black pepper | |

## ASPARAGUS ALMONDINE

SERVES
4

| INGREDIENTS | DIRECTIONS |
|---|---|
| 2 pounds fresh, cooked asparagus | Steam asparagus to al dente, then drain. |
| 2 tablespoons olive oil | Add olive oil to small skillet. |
| ¼ cup slivered almonds | Cook almonds over low heat until golden brown (about 5 to 7 minutes); stir constantly. |
| 1 tablespoon lemon juice | Remove from heat. |
| 1 teaspoon sea salt | Add lemon juice and salt. |
| | Pour over hot asparagus. |

## CRISPY KALE CHIPS

| INGREDIENTS | DIRECTIONS |
|---|---|
| 1 head washed, thoroughly dried kale | Preheat oven to 275°F. |
| 2 tablespoons extra-virgin olive oil | Remove the ribs from the kale and cut into 1 1/2" pieces. |
| Sea salt for sprinkling | Lay on a baking sheet and toss with olive oil and salt. |
| | Bake 10–20 minutes until crisp, turning leaves halfway through. Watch closely. |

# HIGH-FIBER STARCH SIDE DISHES

## SMASHED SWEET POTATOES

SERVES 4

| INGREDIENTS | DIRECTIONS |
|---|---|
| 2 sweet potatoes | Peel and dice sweet potatoes, sauté in oil until very soft and smash. |
| 2 tablespoons olive or coconut oil | Add cinnamon and sea salt. |
| 1 teaspoon cinnamon | Garnish with cinnamon sticks. For a variation, replace the cinnamon with 1 teaspoon basil, 1 teaspoon rosemary and 1/2 teaspoon freshly cracked black pepper. |
| 1/2 teaspoon sea salt | |

## SPICY INDIAN DAHL

SERVES 2

| INGREDIENTS | DIRECTIONS |
|---|---|
| 2 minced cloves garlic | In a large pot, sweat the garlic in the olive oil with the bay leaves on medium heat. |
| 1 teaspoon olive oil | Add in the lentils and coat with the oil. |
| 2 bay leaves | Add in the stock and spices and bring to a boil. |
| 1 cup washed, strained light lentils | Reduce to a low boil and allow to cook about 20 minutes, until the lentils are very soft. |
| 2 cups veggie or chicken stock | |
| 1 teaspoon cumin | |
| 1 teaspoon curry powder | |
| 1/2 teaspoon turmeric | |

## JJ'S FAST BLACK BEANS

SERVES
4

### INGREDIENTS

1 (15-ounce) can black beans

1 (4-ounce) can diced
green chilies

1 teaspoon Mexican seasoning
spice or to taste

### DIRECTIONS

Combine all ingredients in saucepan and warm
over medium heat, stirring occasionally until
heated through.

### TRY THESE VARIATIONS

**Side dish:**
Add salsa on top before serving.

**Dip:**
Puree in food processor. For a colorful appetizer,
layer with guacamole, top with salsa and serve
with crudités.

**Soup:**
Reserve half of the mixture. To the other half,
add ½ cup chicken broth and puree. Add reserved
whole beans. Top with avocado slices and
1 tablespoon salsa.

## SWEET POTATO CHIPS

SERVES
4

### INGREDIENTS

2 sweet potatoes

1 teaspoon cinnamon

1 teaspoon chili powder

1 teaspoon curcumin

1 teaspoon sea salt

### DIRECTIONS

Heat oven to 375°F.

Peel the sweet potatoes and slice them very thin
with either a potato peeler or mandolin.

Spread the potato slices on two baking sheets lined
with parchment paper.

Sprinkle with the cinnamon, chili powder, curcumin
and salt.

Cook about 12 minutes, until golden and crisp.

## SWEET POTATO FRIES

SERVES
(4)

| INGREDIENTS | DIRECTIONS |
|---|---|
| 2 washed, skin-on, medium sweet potatoes, cut into ½" x 1½" strips | Preheat oven to 400 to 420°F. In a bowl, toss the sweet potatoes, oil, sea salt and paprika. |
| 1½ tablespoons coconut or palm fruit oil | Place strips on a greased baking sheet and bake for 20 to 28 minutes, depending on consistency desired. Flip/toss the fries about every 5 to 6 minutes to cook evenly. |
| 1 teaspoon sea salt | |
| 1 teaspoon paprika | |

## EASY QUINOA

| INGREDIENTS | DIRECTIONS |
|---|---|
| 1 cup quinoa | Put quinoa, broth and salt in 2-quart cooking pot and bring to a boil. Cover with a tight-fitting lid and turn the heat down to simmer. |
| 1½ cups veggie or chicken broth | Cook for 15 minutes. Remove quinoa from heat and allow to sit 5 minutes with the lid on. |
| 1 teaspoon sea salt (optional) | Fluff quinoa gently with a fork and serve. |

**OPTIONAL**

Toast quinoa by sautéing over medium heat in 1 tablespoon coconut, palm fruit or olive oil for 5 minutes. Then, add broth and sea salt and cook as directed.

# PROTEIN DISHES

Be sure to add a side salad or veggie dish with these recipes. If the recipe doesn't already include a starchy carb, you can add a high-fiber starchy carb side as well. I like to double these recipes so I can enjoy them again the next day on my salad at lunch.

Portion sizes are approximate here, as they will vary based on your specific protein needs. See page 240 for those guidelines.

## JJ'S HERB-RUBBED PORK TENDERLOIN ROAST

SERVES
4
OR MORE

### INGREDIENTS

½ cup fresh basil

½ cup fresh rosemary

2 tablespoons olive oil

4 cloves garlic

1 teaspoon sage

1 teaspoon thyme

1 teaspoon sea salt

1 teaspoon freshly cracked
black pepper

2 pounds organic pork
tenderloin roast

### DIRECTIONS

Preheat oven to 325°F.

Combine all ingredients except pork tenderloin in
a blender or food processor to create herb blend.

Open pork roast and rub ⅓ herb blend inside.
Wrap back up, tie with cooking string and place
in roasting pan.

Rub remaining herb blend on the outside
of the roast.

Roast for approximately 35 minutes, until internal
temperature reaches 150 to 160 degrees.

This recipe makes great leftovers!

## BASIC CHICKEN PREP

SERVES
2

Preparation time: 20 minutes

### INGREDIENTS

2 (4- to 6-ounce) chicken breasts

Seasoning to taste (freshly
cracked black pepper, lemon
pepper, sea salt, thyme, oregano
or other poultry seasoning)

1 tablespoon olive, palm fruit
or coconut oil

### DIRECTIONS

Preheat oven to 350°F. Clean and rinse the chicken
breasts. Rub exterior of breast with seasoning, such
as black pepper, lemon pepper, sea salt,
thyme, oregano or other poultry seasoning.

Heat a sauté pan or skillet to medium heat and
put oil in the pan. When pan or skillet is hot, place
chicken breasts in pan just long enough to turn
the outside golden brown, then flip over and move
entire pan into the oven to finish cooking, about 8 to
12 minutes. (If your pan isn't oven-resistant, preheat
a cookie sheet or roasting pan and transfer chicken
breasts to it.) Chicken breasts are done when they
are firm to touch and if, when pierced or sliced, their
juice runs clear.

This method can also be used for fish, turkey breasts
and steak.

## LEMON-OREGANO BAKED SOLE

SERVES

**4**

### INGREDIENTS

2 tablespoons lemon juice

1 tablespoon extra-virgin olive oil

2 minced cloves garlic

2 teaspoons chopped oregano

1 teaspoon lemon zest

4 (6-ounce) sole fillets

### DIRECTIONS

Preheat the oven to 350°F.

Mix together the lemon juice, olive oil, garlic, oregano and lemon zest.

Coat the fish evenly with this mix in a baking dish.

Bake for about 17 minutes, until cooked through.

## TURKEY BOLOGNESE OVER QUINOA PASTA

SERVES

**4**

### INGREDIENTS

Sea salt, divided

1 package (16-ounce) quinoa pasta*

1 tablespoon + 1 teaspoon
 extra-virgin olive oil, divided

1 diced, small white onion

5 minced cloves garlic

1 pound ground, organic turkey

1 jar crushed, organic tomatoes

½ cup organic chicken stock

¼ cup organic tomato paste

1 teaspoon chili flakes

1 teaspoon chopped, fresh thyme

1 teaspoon chopped,
fresh oregano

2 tablespoons chopped, fresh basil

Freshly cracked black pepper
to taste

### DIRECTIONS

**Fill a large pot:**

With water and cover. Heat on high to develop a rolling boil. Season the water with a pinch of good sea salt. When the water is boiling, add the pasta and cook until al dente, usually at least 12 minutes. Strain pasta and put back in the pot. Drizzle the hot pasta with 1 teaspoon olive oil and mix to keep the pasta from sticking to itself.

**While the pasta is cooking:**

Heat 1 tablespoon olive oil on medium heat in a large pan. Add the onions and garlic and sweat until translucent. Add the turkey and brown. Add the remaining ingredients except the basil and mix well. Bring to a gentle simmer and allow to reduce about 30 minutes. After reducing, add the basil. Season lightly with sea salt and pepper to taste. Top the cooked pasta with the sauce and serve.

This sauce works great with almost any ground meat. Substitute ground bison for the ground turkey. It's awesome!

* Spirals work well. Look for quinoa flour as the main or only ingredient.

## CHILI-LIME GRILLED CHICKEN SKEWERS

SERVES
4

### INGREDIENTS

¼ cup lime juice

2 tablespoons extra-virgin olive oil

2 teaspoons chopped cilantro

1 teaspoon red pepper flakes

1 teaspoon orange zest

4 large, organic, free-range chicken breasts, sliced ½" thick

12 wooden skewers, soaked in water at least 30 minutes

### DIRECTIONS

In a medium bowl, mix together the lime juice, olive oil, cilantro, red pepper flakes and orange zest.

Dress the raw chicken with this mix until all sides are covered.

Skewer the chicken lengthwise, like threading a needle.

On a clean grill, grill the chicken on medium heat about 5 to 6 minutes per side, until cooked through.

## CHICKEN CACCIATORE

SERVES
2

### INGREDIENTS

2 halved, skinless chicken breasts

Freshly cracked black pepper to taste

1 tablespoon + 1 teaspoon olive oil, divided

1 cup diced onion

8 ounces sliced mushrooms

1½ teaspoons chopped, fresh basil (or dried)

1 teaspoon fresh sage (or dried)

1 bay leaf

¾ cup organic chicken broth

½ cup balsamic vinegar

¼ cup tomato paste

2 minced cloves garlic

### DIRECTIONS

Season chicken breasts with black pepper and sauté in 1 teaspoon olive oil until golden brown on both sides.

Remove chicken and set aside.

Reduce the heat and add to pan the remaining olive oil, onion, mushrooms, basil, sage and bay leaf.

Sauté 5 to 7 minutes.

Add chicken broth, balsamic vinegar, tomato paste and garlic, and simmer 5 to 7 minutes.

Put chicken back in and cook for 5 minutes.

Serve over ½ cup of steamed brown rice, quinoa or brown rice pasta.

## LEMON PICCATA TURKEY TENDERLOIN

SERVES
(2)

This is a great variation on the traditional chicken dish and it gives turkey a great flavor boost!

### INGREDIENTS

Approximately 1 pound of turkey breast cutlets

#### MARINADE INGREDIENTS

1 ¼ cups white wine, divided

¼ cup + 1 tablespoon fresh lemon juice, divided

2 teaspoons sea salt, divided

#### SAUCE INGREDIENTS

2 tablespoons olive oil

Freshly ground cracked black pepper to taste

1 tablespoon finely chopped parsley

1 tablespoon capers

### DIRECTIONS

**Flatten** the turkey breast cutlets to about ¼" thick. You can use a meat hammer or pounder if you have one. Marinade for 12 to 24 hours in 1 cup white wine, ¼ cup lemon juice and 1 teaspoon sea salt.

**Heat** the olive oil in a sauté pan over medium-high heat and sauté the cutlets for 1 to 2 minutes on each side, until lightly browned and cooked through (will vary with thickness of cutlets). Remove and cover with foil or lid to keep warm.

**Deglaze** the pan with the ¼ cup white wine and 1 tablespoon lemon juice, loosening all the browned bits stuck to the pan. Bring to a boil. Season with 1 teaspoon salt and pepper and add the parsley and capers. Add turkey to sauce mixture and serve.

## HERB-CRUSTED CHICKEN BREASTS

SERVES
(4)

### INGREDIENTS

2 cloves garlic

1 tablespoon fresh rosemary

1 tablespoon fresh basil

1 tablespoon extra-virgin olive oil

1 teaspoon sea salt

½ teaspoon freshly cracked black pepper

4 skinless chicken breasts

### DIRECTIONS

Combine herbs, olive oil, salt and pepper in food processor until it becomes a paste.

Spread paste on chicken breasts and cover in refrigerator overnight.

Then, prepare according to the second paragraph of the Basic Chicken Prep directions on page 274.

# SPAGHETTI SQUASH "PASTA" WITH MEAT SAUCE

SERVES
2
OR MORE

Yes, there really is such thing as guilt-free pasta! I promise you won't even miss the noodles, and neither will your thighs.

## INGREDIENTS

1 spaghetti squash

1 chopped onion

1 chopped red bell pepper

2 minced cloves garlic

1 pound ground, lean beef or turkey

1 large jar organic marinara sauce

2 teaspoons Italian seasoning blend

### FOR FUN VARIATIONS

Add chopped sundried tomatoes packed in olive oil (drained), sautéed mushrooms, sliced olives and/or quartered artichoke hearts.

## DIRECTIONS

You can bake or boil the spaghetti squash to get it ready to be your "pasta":

**To bake it:** Preheat oven to 375°F. Pierce the shell several times with a large fork and place in baking dish. Cook squash approximately 1 hour, until flesh is tender.

**To boil it:** Cut squash in half and take out the seeds with a large spoon. Heat a pot of water big enough to hold the squash halves. When the water is boiling, drop the squash in and cook for 15 to 20 minutes, depending on its size. When a fork goes easily into the flesh, the squash is done.

**Whether you bake it or boil it,** let it cool for 10 to 20 minutes so it will be easier to handle before cutting in half (if it isn't already) and removing the seeds (if you didn't already). Pull a fork lengthwise through the flesh to separate it into long strands.

Sauté onion, red pepper and garlic and set aside. Brown the meat and drain well. Add sautéed vegetables and garlic, marinara sauce and seasoning blend. Simmer for 30 minutes.

Serve 2 cups "pasta" topped with 8 ounces meat sauce.

## TURKEY ROLL-UPS

SERVES
(1)

These make a great appetizer, snack or office/school lunch. Get creative with these!

| INGREDIENTS | DIRECTIONS |
| --- | --- |
| 4 to 6 ounces turkey slices | Lay turkey slice flat. Put a stripe of mustard down the center. Add a slice of tomato and avocado, top with a few spinach leaves and roll up. |
| 1 teaspoon Dijon mustard | |
| Fresh or roasted tomato slices | |
| $\frac{1}{2}$ small, sliced avocado | You can also use roast beef or add just about any veggie or condiment you can think of. I have used goat cheese, chopped nuts, roasted veggies, etc. |
| Spinach leaves | |

## SHRIMP DIJON

SERVES         SERVES
(4)  OR  (8)
MEALS      APPETIZERS

### INGREDIENTS

2 pounds peeled, deveined, 21 to 40 size shrimp and/or wild scallops

1 julienned red bell pepper

$\frac{1}{2}$ cup olive oil, divided

$\frac{1}{4}$ cup finely chopped garlic

2 tablespoons dry sherry

1 cup marinara sauce

1 cup Dijon mustard

$\frac{1}{4}$ cup finely chopped, fresh basil

### DIRECTIONS

Marinate the shrimp and bell pepper overnight in $\frac{1}{4}$ cup olive oil and the chopped garlic. Remove the shrimp from the marinade and set aside.

In a large sauté pan over medium-high heat, sauté the bell pepper and marinade for 2 to 3 minutes (add 1 to 2 tablespoons more of olive oil if needed), then add the shrimp. Cook on one side, turn shrimp and sauté until cooked through. Remove shrimp from pan. *Note:* If you are using scallops and shrimp, cook the scallops first because they take slightly longer to cook, then add the shrimp. (I cook the scallops in oil with the red pepper.) Do not overcook.

Deglaze the pan by adding the sherry and scraping up any stuck bits. Over medium heat, add the marinara sauce and Dijon mustard and whisk until blended and smooth. Add the basil and slowly drizzle in $\frac{1}{4}$ cup olive oil while whisking. Whisk and simmer until sauce is slightly reduced, thick and smooth. Add the shrimp mixture back in.

Serve as an appetizer or over sautéed spinach, brown rice or multigrain angel-hair pasta as a main dish. These get gobbled up quickly!

## DIJON-ROSEMARY CRUSTED RACK OF LAMB

SERVES
2
OR MORE

### INGREDIENTS

2 tablespoons Dijon mustard

2 tablespoons dried rosemary, crushed in mortar

2 minced cloves garlic

1 teaspoon sea salt

½ teaspoon freshly cracked black pepper

Rack of lamb

1 teaspoon olive oil

### DIRECTIONS

Combine mustard, rosemary, garlic, salt and pepper into a paste and smear to cover rack of lamb completely. Let sit for 4 to 24 hours in refrigerator to let the flavors marry.

Preheat oven to 500°F. Place rack of lamb in a 12" x 8" x 2" baking dish coated with olive oil. Roast uncovered for 4 minutes. Reduce heat to 350°F, and bake an additional 15 minutes or until a meat thermometer inserted in rack registers 180°F.

## BISTRO SALMON

SERVES
4

### INGREDIENTS

¾ cup lemon juice

1 tablespoon Dijon mustard

1 cup extra-virgin olive oil

4 ounces sundried tomatoes

4 ounces pitted kalamata olives

1 tablespoon capers

1 teaspoon sea salt

½ teaspoon freshly cracked black pepper

4 (6- to 8-ounce) salmon fillets

### DIRECTIONS

Whisk together lemon juice and Dijon mustard, then add olive oil. Add tomatoes, olives, capers, salt and pepper.

Arrange salmon fillets in a baking dish and pour sauce over top. Bake at 400°F for 8 to 10 minutes.

## JJ'S SOUTHWESTERN TURKEY BURGERS

SERVES
4

### INGREDIENTS

1 cup total of chopped red bell pepper and chopped onion

2 ounces diced green chilies

1 tablespoon olive oil

1 teaspoon oregano

Sea salt and freshly cracked black pepper to taste

1 pound ground, lean turkey

### DIRECTIONS

Sauté peppers, onions and green chilies in olive oil. Add oregano, sea salt and black pepper. Add this mixture to the ground turkey and form into 4 patties. Sauté in olive oil, turning gently to avoid breaking apart.

# DESSERTS

## COCONUT ICE CREAM*

### INGREDIENTS

1 cup unsweetened, shredded coconut

3 cups canned, full-fat coconut milk (*not* light)**

$3/4$ cup xylitol

1 teaspoon almond extract

### DIRECTIONS

Unsweetened coconut is very dry, so a few hours before you prepare the ice cream, reconstitute with just a little bit of the coconut milk to soften for a few hours.

Whisk the remaining coconut milk with the xylitol and almond extract. Add to your ice cream maker and follow the manufacturer's directions. When done, stir in the shredded coconut. Your ice cream will be very soft at this point. Put in a covered container and into your freezer to temper/harden if you can stand it, but it is sooo good right from the ice cream maker!

* This treat is really high-calorie, so don't overdo it. A $1/2$ cup serving counts as 2 servings of fat.
** If you use light coconut milk or So Delicious from the carton, your ice cream will be softer and will harden in the freezer more like ice milk, not as creamy smooth.

## RASPBERRY SAUCE ON FRUIT MEDLEY

SERVES
4

### INGREDIENTS

1 cup frozen organic raspberries, defrosted

1 tablespoon light coconut milk

1 to 2 teaspoons xylitol

4 cups chopped fruit in season (e.g., nectarines, peaches, melons)

4 teaspoons unsweetened, shredded coconut

### DIRECTIONS

Blend raspberries, coconut milk and xylitol until smooth. Put 1 cup chopped fruit in a parfait glass and top with 2 tablespoons of raspberry sauce and 1 teaspoon unsweetened, shredded coconut.

### OPTIONS

Top with shaved dark chocolate, toasted almond slices or pecans.

## VIRGIN DIET PIE CRUST

### INGREDIENTS

1 ½ cups almond meal/flour (e.g., Bob's Red Mill)

1 teaspoon xylitol (add more if sweeter crust is desired)

¼ teaspoon sea salt (optional)

3 tablespoons coconut oil

½ teaspoon vanilla

### DIRECTIONS

Preheat oven to 350°F. Mix dry ingredients in a bowl. Add coconut oil and vanilla and stir until thoroughly combined. Press into a 9" pie pan and bake for 10 to 12 minutes, until crust begins to lightly brown. Cool completely before filling.

## BAKED APPLES

SERVES
2

### INGREDIENTS

2 washed, large baking apples (e.g., Rome Beauty, Golden Delicious)

¼ cup xylitol

¼ cup chopped pecans

1 teaspoon cinnamon

1 tablespoon ghee

¾ cup boiling water

### DIRECTIONS

Preheat oven to 375°F. Remove apple cores to ½" of the bottom of the apples using an apple corer or paring knife. Use a spoon to dig out the seeds. Make the holes about ¾" to 1" wide.

In a small bowl, combine the xylitol, pecans and cinnamon. Place apples in an 8" square baking pan. Stuff each apple with this mixture. Top with a dot of ghee.

Add boiling water to the baking pan. Bake 30 to 40 minutes, until tender but not mushy. Remove from the oven and baste the apples several times with the pan juices.

## WARM "PB & J"

SERVES

1

### INGREDIENTS

1 cup frozen berries (any type) and/or dark cherries

1 tablespoon coconut milk

½ teaspoon cinnamon

1 to 2 tablespoons tree nut butter

### DIRECTIONS

Warm berries/cherries and coconut milk over medium heat until fruit is warm. Add cinnamon. Swirl in nut butter.

This dessert is totally decadent.

## NUTTY BARS

Serving size is a 1" x 2" rectangle.

### INGREDIENTS

1 cup room temperature or slightly warmed nut butter

2 scoops vanilla vegan protein powder

2 teaspoons cinnamon

2 cups mixed raw nuts (walnuts, pecans, almonds)

½ cup unsweetened, shredded coconut

### DIRECTIONS

Combine nut butter, vanilla vegan protein powder and cinnamon and stir until thoroughly mixed. Add nuts and coconut and put into baking pan. Cover and refrigerate.

## HEALTHY NUTELLA

SERVES

1

### INGREDIENTS

1 tablespoon water

2 tablespoons chocolate vegan protein powder

1 tablespoon nut butter

### DIRECTIONS

Stir water into chocolate vegan protein powder until it looks like chocolate sauce.

Mix in nut butter.

Enjoy on apple slices.

# RECIPES FOR CYCLE 2: REINTRODUCTION

I created these as single servings. If you want to make these for your family, just increase the ingredients accordingly.

## WEEK 1: GLUTEN CHALLENGE MEALS

### PASTA PRIMAVERA

**INGREDIENTS**

1 cup mixed vegetables (mushrooms, red bell pepper, onion, zucchini, asparagus)

2 tablespoons olive oil

2 tablespoons chopped basil

½ to 1 cup cooked whole-wheat pasta

4 to 8 ounces cooked bay shrimp

2 cups spinach salad

Lemon juice

**DIRECTIONS**

Sauté the vegetables in the olive oil and mix in the basil. Toss with the cooked pasta and top with the shrimp. Squeeze some lemon on the spinach salad and serve alongside the pasta.

### ROASTED VEGETABLE STUFFED PITA

**INGREDIENTS**

1 cup diced vegetables (zucchini, bell pepper, eggplant, onion)

1 tablespoon olive oil

½ to 1 diced clove garlic

½ teaspoon sea salt

1 whole-wheat pita

4 to 8 ounces roasted chicken breast

**DIRECTIONS**

Preheat oven to 375°F. Toss the vegetables in olive oil, garlic and sea salt and roast for 20 to 40 minutes depending on how thick you cut them. Stuff the pita with the vegetable mixture and chicken breast.

## TURKEY ON WHEAT

| INGREDIENTS | DIRECTIONS |
|---|---|
| 2 slices whole-grain bread | Spread mustard on the bread and arrange the turkey, avocado and lettuce into a sandwich. |
| Mustard | Serve with vegetable sticks: carrots, celery and jicama. |
| 4 to 8 ounces nitrate/hormone-free deli turkey meat or fresh, sliced turkey | |
| ¼ avocado | |
| Bibb lettuce | |

## ANGEL-HAIR PASTA WITH TOMATO AND BASIL

| INGREDIENTS | DIRECTIONS |
|---|---|
| 4 to 6 large scallops or 6 to 8 medium ones | Sauté the scallops and tomatoes in garlic and olive oil until the scallops are cooked through, turning once. Remove from heat and add the basil leaves. Pour over the pasta. Serve with the salad. |
| 2 Roma tomatoes | |
| ½ clove garlic | |
| 1 tablespoon olive oil | |
| Fresh, torn basil leaves | |
| ½ to 1 cup cooked angel-hair pasta | |
| 2 cups mixed green salad with balsamic vinaigrette | |

# WEEK 2: SOY CHALLENGE MEALS

## MISO SOUP

**INGREDIENTS**

Miso soup (buy base at the grocery store;
see the Resources section on my website)

1 chopped green onion

4 to 8 ounces cubed tofu

Assorted vegetable sticks

Hummus

**DIRECTIONS**

Add the onion and the tofu to
the soup and serve with the
vegetable sticks and hummus.

## BOCA BURGER WRAPS

**INGREDIENTS**

2 BOCA burgers or another soy-based,
gluten-free burger

Gluten-free mustard

4 thick slices tomato

Sliced avocado

Large leaves of romaine, butter or Bibb lettuce

**DIRECTIONS**

Heat the burgers as directed.
Spread mustard on the burgers,
put a tomato slice on the top and
bottom of each, top with avocado
and wrap with leaves of lettuce.

## LETTUCE WRAPS

**INGREDIENTS**

1 cup total of sliced mushrooms, bean sprouts,
sliced water chestnuts and diced red pepper

4 to 8 ounces tofu

2 tablespoons sesame oil

1 tablespoon tamari or other gluten-free soy sauce

1 tablespoon chopped almonds

Large lettuce leaves (e.g., butter lettuce)

**DIRECTIONS**

Sauté the vegetables and tofu
in the sesame oil and add soy
sauce at the end. Top with
chopped almonds. Wrap in
the lettuce leaves.

## ASIAN CHICKEN SALAD

### INGREDIENTS

2 cups cabbage and romaine mix

4 to 8 ounces chicken strips

$1/2$ cup edamame

1 or 2 diced green onions

1 tablespoon slivered almonds

### DRESSING

1 tablespoon sesame oil

1 tablespoon rice wine vinegar

Sea salt to taste

Freshly ground black pepper to taste

Stevia to taste

### DIRECTIONS

Arrange the first 5 ingredients into a salad. Mix the remaining ingredients together and toss with the salad.

# WEEK 3: EGG CHALLENGE MEALS

## VEGETABLE FRITTATA

### INGREDIENTS

1 cup total of diced asparagus, mushrooms, onions and red pepper

3 tablespoons olive oil

3 eggs

Sliced tomatoes

### DIRECTIONS

Sauté the vegetables in olive oil and pour in beaten eggs. Cover and cook on low heat until done. Or scramble the eggs and vegetables in the olive oil. Serve with sliced tomatoes.

## MIXED GREENS SALAD

### INGREDIENTS

2 cups mixed greens

1 cup assorted sliced cucumber, carrots, scallions and red pepper

4 ounces turkey

2 sliced, boiled eggs

1/3 cup garbanzo beans

1/4 avocado

1 tablespoon extra-virgin olive oil

Lemon juice

### DIRECTIONS

Mix the first 6 ingredients together and toss with the olive oil and lemon juice.

## HOT CEREAL

### INGREDIENTS

1/2 cup cooked buckwheat,* steel-cut oatmeal or amaranth

1/2 cup coconut milk

1/4 cup fresh blueberries

1 tablespoon chopped walnuts

1/2 teaspoon cinnamon

2 boiled eggs

### DIRECTIONS

Mix the cooked cereal with the coconut milk, fruit, nuts and cinnamon. Eat with two boiled eggs.

*Buckwheat is not actually a wheat, and it does not contain gluten.

## POACHED EGGS

### INGREDIENTS

2 cups greens: spinach, chard or other greens

2 tablespoons olive oil

1 sliced heirloom or beefsteak tomato

2 or 3 poached eggs

### DIRECTIONS

Sauté the greens in the olive oil, place on plate. Top with sliced tomatoes and then poached eggs.

# WEEK 4: DAIRY CHALLENGE MEALS

## COTTAGE CHEESE AND FRUIT

**INGREDIENTS**

1 cup low-fat, organic cottage cheese

½ cup chopped apple

1 tablespoon walnut pieces

½ teaspoon cinnamon

Crudités

2 or 3 tablespoons hummus

**DIRECTIONS**

Top the cottage cheese with apples, walnuts and cinnamon.

Serve with crudités and hummus.

## BLACK BEAN SOUP

**INGREDIENTS**

1 cup cooked black bean soup

1 chopped green onion

2 ounces shredded, organic mozzarella

2 cups spinach

4 ounces sliced, roasted chicken

½ cup fresh, sliced mushrooms and julienned red peppers

Extra-virgin olive oil vinaigrette

**DIRECTIONS**

Top the soup with the onion and mozzarella and serve.

Toss the remaining ingredients to create a salad.

## KEFIR SHAKE

Prepare a Virgin Diet Shake using 1 cup low-fat, plain, organic kefir instead of water or coconut milk.

## GREEK-STYLE YOGURT

### INGREDIENTS

6 ounces plain, organic, Greek-style yogurt

1 cup fresh, organic strawberries

2 tablespoons chopped almonds

1 cup chopped, raw cucumber, zucchini
and red pepper

### DIRECTIONS

Mix the fruit and nuts into
the yogurt and serve with the
raw vegetables.

# RECIPES FOR CYCLE 3: THE VIRGIN DIET FOR LIFE

## FLANK STEAK*

SERVES
(2)

This marinade is awesome on any red meat! Flank steak is very lean, which means it can be
a bit tough, so be sure to marinate it for at least 24 hours to help tenderize and flavor it!

### INGREDIENTS

16 ounces flank steak

½ cup wheat-free tamari

¼ cup balsamic vinegar

2 tablespoons
Worcestershire sauce

1 tablespoon dry mustard

2 minced cloves garlic

Freshly cracked black pepper
to taste

### DIRECTIONS

Combine all the ingredients and marinate for
24 hours. Grill or broil until done to your liking.
Slice across the grain into thin slices.

*This recipe is for those of you who are not soy-sensitive.

## JJ'S TEQUILA TREAT

SERVES
(2)

### INGREDIENTS

4 ounces tequila

½ cup freshly squeezed lime juice

¼ cup peeled, seeded, crushed cucumber

2 tablespoons freshly squeezed pink grapefruit juice

1 tablespoon finely chopped basil

### DIRECTIONS

You can serve it over ice or add sparkling mineral water to it.

Although I don't usually believe in food- or drink-based rewards, I treat myself to one of these when I finish large projects, like writing this book!

# READER FAVORITES

In the next section you will find twenty of the best homemade recipes that embrace the principles of the Virgin Diet, submitted by readers who had amazing success after following the plan. These recipes represent hope, perseverance, commitment and transformation. I hope the contributors' stories inspire and motivate you as they have me and countless others, and their delicious recipes delight your taste buds.

## BREAKFAST

KATHY HENDRICKS
Stayton, Oregon

"I have been on the Virgin Diet for about 2 months now. I am feeling really good, going to the gym and exercising for the first time in years. I have way more energy now than I did before. So far, I have lost 15 pounds."

## MIXED BERRY PANCAKES

SERVES

| INGREDIENTS | DIRECTIONS |
|---|---|
| 1 tablespoon ground flaxseed | Make a flax slurry: Mix the flaxseed with water and let stand for 3 to 5 minutes. |
| 3 tablespoons water | |
| 2 scoops Virgin Diet All-in-One Shake Mix* | Meanwhile blend the shake mix, oatmeal, coconut milk and berries in a medium bowl. Add the flax slurry, while stirring to combine. |
| 1/3 cup gluten-free oatmeal | |
| 1/3 cup unsweetened coconut milk | Heat a nonstick skillet over a medium-high heat. Drop the batter into the skillet by the spoonful, so that it forms rounds. Cook until bubbles form, 2 to 3 minutes. Flip and cook an additional 1 to 2 minutes. |
| 1/2 cup mixed berries | |
| Stevia, for dusting | |
| | Serve with a dusting of stevia. |

* Available at jjvirginstore.com

PAULA LEMMO
Middleton, Massachusetts

> "I started the program at the end of January, and in the first 8 weeks,
> I lost about 25 pounds."

## MORNING GLORY OATMEAL

SERVES

### INGREDIENTS

¾ cup gluten-free old-fashioned rolled oats

1 small apple, peeled and chopped

2 tablespoons walnuts, chopped

½ cup water

1 cup coconut milk

2 scoops Virgin Diet All-in-One Chai protein powder

1 teaspoon cinnamon

1 tablespoon organic roasted cacao nibs

¼ cup organic fresh or frozen berries

### DIRECTIONS

Place the oats, apple and walnuts in saucepan over a medium heat. Add the water and cook for 5 to 10 minutes (use more or less water as necessary to reach the desired consistency).

While the oatmeal is cooking, blend the coconut milk, protein powder and cinnamon.

Add the milk mixture to the oatmeal and heat for another 30 to 60 seconds. Remove from heat.

Top with the berries and cacao nibs and serve.

# SALADS

JENNIFER POYNTER
Newhall, California

"Within 3 days, the 33 years of stomach issues were gone. *I feel nothing? No gremlins eating away at my insides?* I've lost 10 pounds in less than three weeks. This isn't a diet; diets make us feel anxious and hungry. This makes you feel peaceful."

## SPRING SALAD

SERVES
2

### INGREDIENTS

10 asparagus spears, trimmed

1 cup haricot verts, trimmed

2 tablespoons lemon juice

2 teaspoons ginger, grated

2 teaspoons shallot, minced

1/4 cup extra virgin olive oil

Salt and pepper to taste

1 pinch xylitol

6-ounce cooked free-range chicken breast, cut into bite-size pieces

4 cups mixed baby greens

1/2 cup raspberries

2 scallions, chopped

### DIRECTIONS

Bring a large pot of water to a boil. Add the asparagus and haricot verts and blanch for 1 to 2 minutes, until they are bright green and crisp-tender. Drain and plunge them into a bowl of ice water to stop the cooking process.

In a small bowl, mix the lemon juice, ginger and shallot. Slowly whisk in the oil and season with salt, pepper and xylitol.

Remove the asparagus and haricot verts from the ice bath, chop into 1" pieces and place in a large bowl. Add the chopped chicken and mix well.

Gently stir in the baby greens, raspberries and scallions.

Drizzle with the dressing, tossing gently to coat all the ingredients, and serve.

**DEBBIE BANEY**
Mesa, Arizona

"My husband and I started the diet on April 12 with a kickoff
party for a group of us who wanted to do this together. I have suffered
my entire life with weight, energy, allergies, foggy brain,
constipation, and infertility issues. It is now June, and I am delighted
to say that I have lost 19 pounds so far. My energy is increasing,
my allergies are decreasing, and the "fog" in my brain has lifted!"

## HEARTY LENTIL LUNCHEON SALAD

SERVES

### INGREDIENTS

1 (15-ounce) can lentils, rinsed
and drained

3 to 4 cups romaine-baby spring
mix

1 (5-ounce) can of tuna or
salmon, drained

1 avocado, diced

1 stalk celery, chopped

¼ cup onion, chopped

1 teaspoon Italian seasoning

6 cherry tomatoes, chopped

### DIRECTIONS

Heat the lentils in a saucepan over medium heat
until warmed through, 3 to 5 minutes.

Line each of two bowls with the lettuce.

In another bowl, gently mix the tuna, avocado, celery,
onion and seasoning.

Lay the lentils onto the lettuce and top with a mound
of the tuna mixture.

Garnish with the tomatoes and serve.

CATHY BOUCHER
Lowell, Massachusetts

"Before beginning the Virgin Diet, I had no energy, joint pain,
and constant congestion. I felt so much older, and I thought I *looked*
older than my 53 years. After seven weeks, I had lost 20 pounds.
The joint pain and congestion were gone, and I had so much more energy.
I also found out that I was dairy intolerant. The Virgin Diet is so much
more than a diet to me. It has become a way of life."

# PROVENÇAL BEAN SALAD

SERVES
4
OR MORE

### INGREDIENTS

1 (15-ounce) can red kidney beans, rinsed and drained

1 (15-ounce) can black beans, rinsed and drained

1 (15-ounce) can garbanzo beans, rinsed and drained

1 red onion, diced

1 small red pepper, chopped

1 celery rib, diced

¼ cup fresh cilantro, chopped

3 tablespoons white balsamic vinegar

2 tablespoons Greek extra-virgin olive oil

2 tablespoons lemon juice

1 tablespoon whole-grain mustard

1 tablespoon Herbes de Provence

1 teaspoon sea salt

Cracked fresh pepper to taste

### DIRECTIONS

Combine the beans, onion, red pepper, celery and cilantro in a medium bowl.

In a small bowl, whisk the vinegar, oil, lemon juice, mustard, Herbes de Provence, salt and pepper. Pour the dressing over the bean mixture and toss well to coat.

Cover and refrigerate for at least an hour before serving.

# SOUPS

ALYSON SLUTZKY
Maplewood, New Jersey

"I've lost about 17 pounds, and my digestion has improved
tremendously. I feel better about my body, and I've had a great
time buying new clothes. I'm no longer self-conscious about the way
I look. I'm *enjoying* eating nourishing food."

## GAZPACHO

SERVES (2)

### INGREDIENTS

1 garlic clove, minced

¼ medium onion, cut into 1"
pieces

1 medium cucumber, halved,
seeded and cut into 1" pieces

2 plum tomatoes, cut into 1"
pieces

3 cups tomato juice

¼ cup white wine vinegar

1 teaspoon salt

¼ teaspoon black pepper,
coarse ground

### DIRECTIONS

Place the garlic, onion, cucumber and tomatoes in
a food processor and pulse until they are coarsely
chopped. Transfer the chopped vegetables into a
large bowl.

Add the tomato juice, vinegar, salt and pepper, then
mix well.

Cover and refrigerate for at least 30 minutes before
serving.

CYNTHIA KNIGHT
Kernersville, North Carolina

"In the past 6 months, I have lost 18 pounds, and my husband has lost
26 pounds. He has been able to exercise more (since I have been dealing
with a pinched nerve in my neck), but we both have experienced a boost
in energy, and I have seen greatly reduced inflammation in my joints.
We both need to have our wedding bands resized!! Even if I never lose
another pound, I will continue to eat according to JJ's book,
just because I feel so much better."

## TARRAGON SOUP

SERVES
4
OR MORE

### INGREDIENTS

1 pound ground grass-fed beef
or 1 pound ground free-range
chicken

2 ½ to 3 cups chopped onion

7 to 8 celery stalks, chopped

2 small cloves garlic, crushed

2 quarts organic chicken or
vegetable broth

3 cups water

3 (15-ounce) cans great Northern
beans, rinsed and drained

2 (14.5-ounce) cans organic
tomatoes, chopped

2 tablespoons fresh tarragon

2 tablespoons fresh basil

1 ½ teaspoons fresh oregano

Salt and pepper to taste

### DIRECTIONS

Brown the ground meat in a large soup pot, breaking
up the large chunks with a wooden spoon.

Add the onion, celery and garlic. Stir and cook for
3 to 5 minutes.

Add the broth and water. Bring to a boil, reduce the
heat to medium and cook for 1 hour.

Add the beans, tomatoes, tarragon, basil and oregano.
Stir to combine, reduce the heat and simmer for at
least another hour, stirring occasionally.

Season to taste with salt and pepper and serve.

# SIDE DISHES

DAWN WARD
Knoxville, Tennessee

"During Cycle 1, my energy level increased, my brain fog decreased and my overall drive for life has returned. I am so pleased that I don't even *want* to reintroduce the seven high-FI foods back into my diet."

## MEXICAN QUINOA

SERVES
2
OR MORE

### INGREDIENTS

2 cups vegetable broth

1 cup quinoa, rinsed

1 tablespoon coconut oil

1 small onion, chopped

1 cup mushrooms, sliced

1 (14-ounce) can diced tomatoes with green peppers and garlic

2 chipotle peppers in adobo sauce, chopped (reserve the rest of the can for another use)

### DIRECTIONS

Bring the vegetable broth and quinoa to a boil. Cover, reduce the heat to low and simmer for 15 minutes or until the liquid is absorbed.

Meanwhile heat the oil in large skillet and add the onion and mushrooms. Sauté until the onion is translucent and the mushrooms are browned, 5 to 8 minutes.

Add the tomatoes and the chipotle peppers and cook for an additional 2 minutes.

Remove from the heat and stir in the quinoa. Serve as a side dish or add shrimp or chicken to make it a main course.

ERIC MOORE
Minneapolis, Minnesota

"I am a new person. I no longer have high cholesterol, high blood pressure, heart palpitations, dandruff and skin rashes, joint pain, gassing and bloating after meals or depression and anxiety. I am so thankful to JJ. . . . This diet has changed my life, and it has helped me to help so many other people suffering from chronic fatigue, joint pains, headaches, yeast overgrowth and subclinical depression and anxiety."

## ZUCCHINI NOODLES

SERVES

### INGREDIENTS

SAUCE:

2 tablespoons raw, unsalted almond butter

1 ½ tablespoons lime juice

1 teaspoon sea salt

½ teaspoon minced garlic

½ teaspoon minced fresh ginger

⅛ teaspoon red pepper flakes

1 to 2 tablespoons water

2 to 3 drops liquid stevia, or to taste

ZUCCHINI:

1 organic zucchini, cut into thin ribbons

½ cup diced cucumber

¼ cup chopped carrot

2 to 4 tablespoons chopped fresh cilantro

Optional toppings: sunflower seeds/pumpkin seeds

### DIRECTIONS

Place the almond butter, lime juice, salt, garlic, ginger and red pepper flakes in a blender and process until smooth. With the motor running, add the water slowly, using more or less to reach the desired consistency. Set it aside.

Season with stevia to taste. Set it aside.

For the zucchini noodles: sprinkle the zucchini ribbons with salt and leave them in a colander for 10 minutes. Squeeze out the excess water from the zucchini with a paper towel.

Toss the noodles with the cucumber, carrot and cilantro.

Drizzle the noodles with the sauce, top with the seeds, if using, and serve.

# MAIN DISHES

**BECKY GIGANTI**
Springfield, Illinois

"It was early December that I began the diet, and by January 7, I went from a size 8 to a size 6. My skin began to clear up, and I had a different skin tone—"glowy," someone called it. People ask me daily, 'What have you done to lose so much weight?' I tell them about the Virgin Diet. I tell them that they have to be ready to make the commitment. I was ready, and it has been a life-changer for this girl."

## PISTACHIO AND BROCCOLI PESTO-CRUSTED SALMON

SERVES

### INGREDIENTS

²/₃ cup broccoli florets

²/₃ cup fresh basil leaves

1 tablespoon raw pine nuts

1 teaspoon garlic, minced

2 tablespoons extra-virgin olive oil

1 pinch each salt and pepper

4 (3-ounce) wild salmon fillets

³/₄ cup pistachios, shelled and roughly chopped

4 cups baby spinach

### DIRECTIONS

Preheat the oven to 375°F.

Pulse the broccoli, basil leaves, pine nuts and garlic in a food processor until well blended. With the motor running, drizzle in the olive oil and a bit of water until the consistency is a thick puree.

Spread the pesto on the top of the salmon fillets and sprinkle with the pistachios. Season lightly with salt and pepper.

Bake for 10 to 15 minutes, or until the salmon is opaque and flakes easily with fork.

Place 1 cup baby spinach on each of the four plates. Top with a salmon fillet and serve.

SUSAN ALSTON
Natick, Massachusetts

"Prior to embarking on my new lifestyle, I was overweight, and I suffered from joint aches and pains. I had chronic tendonitis for 8 months, as well as headaches and heartburn. . . . Once I switched to the Virgin Diet, all of my symptoms virtually disappeared in a few weeks, and I started dropping weight and feeling *awesome*. I clearly had a significant sensitivity to gluten. My skin looks better. *I* look better. I have a spring in my step. . . . I *feel* wonderful! It'll cost you though . . . you're going to have to buy smaller clothes!"

## ROASTED VEGGIE BOWL

SERVES
2
OR MORE

| INGREDIENTS | DIRECTIONS |
|---|---|
| 1 red bell pepper, chopped | Toss the vegetables with oil, salt and pepper in a large bowl. Let stand for 30 minutes. |
| 1 yellow bell pepper, chopped | |
| 1 sweet potato, cubed | Preheat the oven to 400°F. |
| 1 onion, chopped | Line a couple of baking sheets with parchment paper and spread the vegetables on them. Roast for 15 to 20 minutes. |
| 1 zucchini, chopped | |
| 8 ounces mushrooms, sliced | |
| 8 asparagus spears, trimmed and cut into 1" pieces | Toss the roasted vegetables with the cooked quinoa, rice and chicken or seaford and serve. |
| 2 tablespoons olive oil | |
| Sea salt and pepper to taste | |
| 1 cup cooked quinoa | |
| 1 cup cooked brown rice | |
| 8 ounces cooked chicken, shrimp, salmon or scallops | |

BONNIE NUNEZ
Long Beach, California

"I lost 5 pounds in the first 2 weeks. My headaches are significantly reduced, which is a *huge* relief after 10-plus years of having constant headaches (80 to 90 percent of the time). . . . I still think that following the Virgin Diet is difficult; however, the health benefits are completely worth it, and it has made a huge difference in my quality of life!"

## COCONUT CURRY CHICKEN

SERVES
4

### INGREDIENTS

1 tablespoon coconut oil

3 boneless, skinless chicken breasts, cut into bite-size pieces

1 small onion, chopped

2 cloves garlic, minced

1 (14-ounce) can coconut milk

2 tablespoons yellow curry powder

2 medium zucchini, chopped

4 medium carrots, chopped

2 bell peppers, chopped

1 cup mushrooms

Optional: red lentils or brown rice, for serving

### DIRECTIONS

Heat the coconut oil in a large skillet over a medium heat, and add the chicken, onion and garlic.

When the chicken is cooked almost all the way through, add the coconut milk and curry powder. Simmer for 2 minutes.

Add the zucchini, carrots and peppers and simmer for 5 to 10 minutes more, or until cooked through.

Add the mushrooms and simmer for 2 minutes more.

Serve over cooked red lentils or brown rice, if desired.

COLEEN WHEELER
Coraopolis, Pennsylvania

"Since starting the Virgin Diet, I am off all of my allergy medication, and I
rarely need to take anything for pain! I have more energy, and my mood is
great! I can't imagine going back to feeling like I did before."

## ASIAN STIR-FRY

SERVES

4

### INGREDIENTS

1 tablespoon red palm oil

1 tablespoon sesame oil

1 onion, chopped

1 cup chopped red pepper

1 cup chopped zucchini

1 cup chopped mushrooms

2 cloves garlic, minced

1 cup cooked chicken, cut into
bite-size pieces

1 cup cooked shrimp, cut into
bite-size pieces

1 cup organic chicken broth

2 tablespoons coconut aminos,
plus more for serving, if desired

1 teaspoon rice wine vinegar

2 teaspoons ginger, freshly
grated

1 teaspoon cumin

1 pinch red pepper flakes

Sea salt and pepper to taste

1 tablespoon brown rice flour
dissolved in ¼ cup of COLD water

1 cup rice noodles rehydrated in
HOT water for 8 minutes then
drained

### DIRECTIONS

Heat the oils in a large skillet or wok over a medium-
high heat.

Add the onion, bell pepper, zucchini, mushrooms
and garlic and stir-fry until the vegetables are
crisp-tender.

Add the chicken and shrimp and toss until they are
heated through.

Add the broth, coconut aminos, rice vinegar, ginger,
cumin and red pepper flakes and bring all to a boil.

Add the dissolved flour, stirring frequently until the
sauce is thickened.

Add the noodles, tossing to coat them in the sauce.
Heat through, for 2 to 3 minutes.

Serve with coconut aminos on the side, if desired.

CAREN FIELDS
Richmond, Virginia

"I have lost 8 pounds in 2 weeks, and better yet, I am getting back
my old energy and zest for life! My husband is thrilled to see his old wife
coming back, but I warned him that I just might be *better than ever*
based on how I am feeling so far!"

## SHRIMP CREOLE

SERVES

4

### INGREDIENTS

1 tablespoon coconut oil

1 cup chopped celery

1 cup chopped onion

1 cup chopped green pepper

1 (6-ounce) can tomato paste

2 bay leaves, crushed

½ teaspoon fish sauce

1 dash Tabasco

1 pound wild-caught shrimp,
peeled and deveined

Salt and pepper to taste

2 cups cooked brown rice

### DIRECTIONS

Heat the oil in skillet over medium heat. Add the
celery, onion and pepper and cook for 3 minutes
or until tender-crisp.

Add the tomato paste, bay leaves, fish sauce, Tabasco
and a couple of tablespoons of water, stirring to
combine. Cover and simmer for about 15 minutes,
stirring occasionally.

Add the shrimp and continue cooking for 3 to
5 minutes until they are pink and cooked through.

Season to taste with salt and pepper.

Serve over a bed of brown rice.

KATELYN RICHARDS

Fort Collins, Colorado

"Before I started the Virgin Diet, I suffered from hormonal problems
and a little extra weight around my stomach. I was missing out on feeling
attractive and living the active lifestyle that I was used to living, because of
fatigue issues. Now I am at my ideal weight, I have more energy and
I don't suffer from hormonal irregularities."

## BAKED SALMON AND ARTICHOKE HEARTS, MUSHROOMS, ASPARAGUS AND PEAS IN LEMON SAUCE

SERVES

### INGREDIENTS

1 bunch asparagus, trimmed and cut into 1" pieces

1 tablespoon olive oil

3 cups canned artichoke hearts, drained

1 cup fresh or frozen peas

²/₃ cups sliced white button mushrooms

¼ cup chicken or vegetable broth

1 tablespoon fresh lemon juice

¹/₃ cup slivered almonds

Salt and pepper to taste

1 cup cooked brown rice

### DIRECTIONS

Steam the asparagus until al dente, 3 to 4 minutes.

Heat the oil in a skillet over medium heat. Add the asparagus, artichoke hearts, peas and mushrooms. Cook for about 2 minutes. Add the broth and lemon juice; bring to a boil.

Reduce the heat to low, cover and simmer until the peas are tender, 10 to 15 minutes for fresh peas and 5 minutes for frozen peas.

Season with salt and pepper.

Remove from the heat and add the almond slivers.

Serve over brown rice.

JUDY LABELLE
Indian Head Park, Illinois

"I am 70 years old. I have dieted most of my adult life. As I got older, losing weight became more difficult. Trying the Virgin Diet was an experiment. I had tried every other diet out there over the years, so why not? I could not believe what happened over the first 3 weeks! I lost weight every day. I continue to lose weight and inches, and I never count calories. . . . I feel great! I am wearing clothes that have not fit for years."

## CARIBBEAN CHICKEN STEW

SERVES
8

### INGREDIENTS

1 1/2 tablespoons olive oil

1 large yellow onion, chopped

1 red, orange, or yellow pepper, diced

3 to 4 large garlic cloves, crushed

1 bay leaf

2 teaspoons cinnamon

1 teaspoon allspice

1 teaspoon nutmeg

1/2 teaspoon cayenne

1 (16-ounce) can no-sugar-added diced tomatoes

2 cups low-sodium chicken broth

1 (15-ounce) can black beans, undrained

1 1/2 pounds poached skinless, boneless chicken breasts, shredded

1 1/2 cups sliced zucchini, cut into thick half moons

Sea salt and freshly ground pepper

### DIRECTIONS

Heat the oil in a large pot over a medium heat.

Add the onion, pepper and garlic and sauté for 3 minutes.

Add the bay leaf, cinnamon, allspice, nutmeg and cayenne and continue cooking for 3 minutes.

Add the tomatoes, broth and beans. Simmer covered for 15 minutes, stirring occasionally.

Add the chicken and zucchini and simmer covered for an additional 10 minutes. Remove bay leaf.

Season to taste with salt and pepper and serve.

KAREN MORRIS
Buffalo Grove, Illinois

"After 24 hours, my eyeaches and headaches vanished. Pimples on
my scalp disappeared, and chocolate cravings faded away. I was energized,
happy, and I never felt better in my whole life. Within 6 weeks, I was
taken off thyroid pills, vitamin D supplements and depression medication.
Blood pressure, blood work, sugar levels and cholesterol levels all
improved drastically. The way I felt inside my "new" body was more
important than the weight loss for me.
I lost 5 pounds the first week and continued to lose a total of
33 pounds in 4 months."

## LUSCIOUS LASAGNA

SERVES

### INGREDIENTS

1 pound ground grass-fed beef

1 (25.5-ounce) Organic Garden vegetable pasta sauce, divided

1 ½ cups diced red pepper

1 cup diced red onion

1 teaspoon garlic salt

1 teaspoon dried oregano

4 brown rice lasagna noodles

1 tablespoon coconut oil

1 cup diced zucchini

1 cup diced broccoli

1 cup diced baby spinach

4 cloves garlic, minced

### DIRECTIONS

Preheat the oven to 350°F.

Brown the beef in a nonstick skillet until it is no longer pink. Drain the excess fat.

Add 1 ½ cups of the pasta sauce, the red pepper, onion, garlic salt and oregano. Set aside.

Bring the water to a boil in a large pot and cook the lasagna noodles according to the package directions. Drain and rinse.

Heat the oil in a skillet and sauté the zucchini, broccoli, baby spinach and garlic until softened, 5 to 8 minutes. Set aside.

Begin layering the lasagna into an 8 x 8" baking pan as follows: 1 cup pasta sauce to cover the bottom of the pan, 2 lasagna noodles, ⅓ of the beef mixture, ½ of the vegetable mixture, 2 lasagna noodles, ⅓ of the beef mixture, ½ of the vegetable mixture, ⅓ of the beef mixture, then the remaining pasta sauce.

Bake in the oven for 35 minutes or until it is hot and bubbly.

Let the lasagna stand for about 5 minutes to allow it to set before serving.

# DESSERTS

**SUSAN MANNING**
Seattle, Washington

"I had spent my entire adult life dieting on and off, and slowly working my way up to an uncomfortable overweight status. I was self-conscious and discouraged, taunted by a closet full of clothes that no longer fit. Even worse, I began to suffer from arthritis in my knees and a slipped disc, and I was often unable to get even the little bit of exercise I had previously attempted.

I've lost 21 pounds, which has greatly impacted my mobility, and it has also enabled me to wear those taunting clothes. (Hey, a whole new wardrobe . . . for free . . . sort of.) I walk several miles a day, and if I am careful, will be able to put off getting new knees indefinitely. I am also less self-conscious, and even department store dressing rooms with 360-degree mirrors are not so terrifying."

## APPLE CHERRY CRUMBLE

SERVES
(4)

### INGREDIENTS

4 large Braeburn or Fuji apples, cut into 1" cubes

1 1/2 cups frozen unsweetened cherries

1 teaspoon lemon juice

2 scoops vanilla protein shake mix

2 scoops chia protein shake mix

1 cup chopped cashews or almonds

1 teaspoon cinnamon

1/4 cup coconut oil, melted

### DIRECTIONS

Preheat the oven to 350°F.

Place the apples, cherries, and lemon juice in an ovenproof casserole dish and stir well.

In a small bowl, mix the protein shake mixes, nuts and cinnamon. Add the coconut oil and cut in with forks until the mixture is crumbly.

Pour the topping over the apple-cherry mixture, covering it completely.

Bake uncovered in an oven for 35 to 40 minutes. If crust begins to brown too early, cover loosely with foil and continue baking.

LEAH NEWSOME
Colerain, North Carolina

"I lost a total of 21 pounds in 10 weeks, and I did it without doing any extra
physical activity whatsoever. I went from a pants size of 8 to a 4 (and even
a 2 in some cases). I am happy with my weight loss, but what totally blows
me away is how much my health and energy level have improved."

# RICE BERRY PUDDING

SERVES

3

## INGREDIENTS

½ cup brown rice

1 ⅓ cups water

1 cup fresh blueberries

½ cup unsweetened coconut milk

3 tablespoons pecans, chopped

2 tablespoons flaxseed, finely ground

1 teaspoon cinnamon

¼ teaspoon sea salt

⅛ teaspoon ground ginger

⅛ teaspoon nutmeg

## DIRECTIONS

Bring the rice and water to the boil, reduce the heat to low, cover and cook for approximately 30 minutes, until rice is tender.

Stir in the remaining ingredients and simmer until heated through and slightly thickened. Serve immediately.

BARBARA DUTTERER
Columbia, Maryland

"I started the Virgin Diet plan on April 22, and something magical
happened. I never felt deprived. I have more energy than I have had in
years, and the weight just seemed to melt off. Thank you, JJ Virgin,
for my new lease on life!!!"

## COCONUT TAPIOCA PUDDING

SERVES

4

### INGREDIENTS

⅓ cup tapioca pearls

2 cups almond milk, divided

1 cup coconut milk

1 teaspoon vanilla extract

Liquid stevia to taste (optional)

1 teaspoon tapioca starch mixed
with 1 teaspoon water

¼ teaspoon sea salt

Toasted coconut chips, for
garnish

### DIRECTIONS

In large glass bowl, mix the tapioca pearls and 1 cup
of the almond milk. Stir, cover and chill for at least
4 hours and up to overnight in the refrigerator.

After the tapioca mixture has chilled, pour it into
a medium saucepan and add the remaining cup of
almond milk.

Bring to a boil over medium heat. Add the coconut
milk, vanilla and stevia, if using, and cook for another
12 to 15 minutes, stirring constantly.

Reduce the heat to low and add the tapioca starch
mixture and salt. Cook, stirring, for an additional
5 minutes. Cool in a glass bowl for at least an hour
before serving.

Serve slightly warm or chilled garnished with toasted
coconut chips.

# APPENDIX A

## The Virgin Diet Shopping List

These are the items that I keep on hand so I can assemble healthy, delicious Virgin Diet meals in minutes!

## FOR YOUR FREEZER

- ☐ Frozen berries (Blueberries, strawberries and raspberries are wonderful.)
- ☐ Frozen shrimp
- ☐ Frozen veggies (Have a wide variety and use them for sides, soups and stir-fry.)
- ☐ Grass-fed beef tenderloin
- ☐ King crab
- ☐ Organic chicken and turkey sausages
- ☐ Organic, free-range chicken and turkey breasts
- ☐ Pasture-fed pork tenderloin
- ☐ Wild fish (My favorites are sole, salmon, scallops and halibut (Alaskan).)

# FOR YOUR FRIDGE

- ☐ Asparagus
- ☐ Broccoli
- ☐ Chia seeds
- ☐ Coconut milk
- ☐ Dijon mustard (gluten-free)
- ☐ Flax seed (Grind fresh before use.)
- ☐ Fresh, low-glycemic index (e.g., berries, apples)
- ☐ Fresh salsa
- ☐ Guacamole
- ☐ Hummus
- ☐ Iced green tea (Make fresh, no sugar added.)
- ☐ Lemons
- ☐ Limes
- ☐ Mushrooms
- ☐ Nut butters (almond, pecan, walnut, macadamia and cashew butter)
- ☐ Organic turkey slices
- ☐ Red onions
- ☐ Red peppers
- ☐ Roast beef slices
- ☐ Roasted whole chicken
- ☐ Salad greens (Look for baby spinach and arugula in tubs.)
- ☐ Sparkling mineral water

# FOR YOUR PANTRY

- ☐ Artichoke hearts
- ☐ Black beans
- ☐ Brown rice
- ☐ Brown rice pasta
- ☐ Coconut milk
- ☐ Diced green chilies
- ☐ Garbanzo beans
- ☐ Green teas (Drink both iced and hot.)
- ☐ Lentils
- ☐ Organic chicken broth
- ☐ Quinoa
- ☐ Quinoa pasta
- ☐ Raw nuts (almonds, cashews, pecans, walnuts, macadamia nuts, Brazil nuts, pistachios)
- ☐ Rice noodles
- ☐ Sun-dried tomatoes in olive oil
- ☐ Thai Kitchen red curry coconut sauce
- ☐ Vinegar (red, balsamic, rice) for salad dressings

## FOR YOUR VEGGIE/FRUIT BIN

Store these in open bins in a dark spot, not in the fridge.

☐ Avocados

☐ Beets

☐ Butternut squash

☐ Garlic

☐ Kabocha squash

☐ Onions

☐ Sweet potatoes

☐ Tomatoes

## KEY OILS

☐ Coconut or palm fruit oil (for high-temperature cooking)

☐ Extra-virgin olive oil (to use raw)

☐ Olive Oil (for medium-temperature cooking)

## SPICES

☐ Basil

☐ Black peppercorn

☐ Cinnamon

☐ Cumin

☐ Curcumin (turmeric)

☐ Herbs de Provence

☐ Italian spice blend

☐ Mexican spice blend

☐ Oregano

☐ Red chile

☐ Red pepper

☐ Rosemary

☐ Sea salt

# APPENDIX B

## Converting to Metrics

| VOLUME MEASUREMENT CONVERSIONS | |
|---|---|
| U.S. | METRIC |
| ¼ teaspoon | 1.25 milliliters |
| ½ teaspoon | 2.5 milliliters |
| ¾ teaspoon | 3.75 milliliters |
| 1 teaspoon | 5 milliliters |
| 1 tablespoon | 15 milliliters |
| ¼ cup | 62.5 milliliters |
| ½ cup | 125 milliliters |
| ¾ cup | 187.5 milliliters |
| 1 cup | 250 milliliters |

| WEIGHT CONVERSION MEASUREMENTS ||
|---|---|
| U.S. | METRIC |
| 1 ounce | 28.4 grams |
| 8 ounces | 227.5 grams |
| 16 ounces (1 pound) | 455 grams |

| COOKING TEMPERATURE CONVERSIONS ||
|---|---|
| Celsius/Centigrade | 0°C and 100°C are arbitrarily placed at the melting and boiling points of water and are standard to the metric system. |
| Fahrenheit | Fahrenheit established 0°F as the stabilized temperature when equal amounts of ice, water and salt are mixed. |

To convert temperatures in Fahrenheit to Celsius, use this formula:

$$C = (F-32) \times 0.5555$$

So, for example, if you are baking at 350°F and want to know that temperature in Celsius, use this calculation:

$$C = (350-32) \times 0.5555 = 176.65°C$$

# SOURCES

1. Nackers, LM, KM Ross, and MG Perri. 2010. The association between rate of initial weight loss and long-term success in obesity treatment: Does slow and steady win the race? *Int J Behav Med.* 17(3):161–67.

2. Sciamanna, CN, et al. 2011. Practices associated with weight loss versus weight-loss maintenance results of a national survey. *Am J Prev Med.* 41(2):159–66.

3. Gislason, S. *The Book of Gluten: Cereal Grains and Gluten Related Diseases.* Vancouver, BC: Environmed Research.

4. Bray, GA. 2000. Afferent signals regulating food intake. *Proc Nutr Soc.* 59(3):373–84.

5. http://pcrm.org/media/news/nutrition-expert-provides-new-ammunition-for-fast

6. Kessler, DA. 2009. *The End of Overeating: Taking Control of the Insatiable American Appetite.* New York: Rodale.

7. Hollis, JF, et al. 2000. Weight loss during the intensive intervention phase of the weight-loss maintenance trial. *Am J Prev Med.* 35(2):118–26.

8. Biesiekierski, JR, et al. 2011. Gluten causes gastrointestinal symptoms in subjects without celiac disease: A double-blind randomized placebo-controlled trial. *Am J Gastroenterol.* 106(3):508–15.

9. Osborne, Peter, audio interview, http://www.glutenfreesociety.org/gluten-free-society-blog/gluten-in-grains-central-to-autoimmune-diseases

10. White, LR, H Petrovich, GW Ross, and KH Masaki. 1996. Association of mid-life consumption of tofu with late life cognitive impairment and dementia: The Honolulu-Asia Aging Study. Paper presented at the fifth International Conference on Alzheimer's Disease, Osaka, Japan.

11. Hogervorst, E, et al. 2008. High tofu intake is associated with worse memory in elderly Indonesian men and women. *Dement Geriatr Cogn Disord.* 26(1):50–57.

12. Barr, SI. 2003. Increased dairy product or calcium intake: Is body weight or composition affected in humans? *J Nutr.* 133(1):245S–248S.

13. Berkey, CS, et al. 2005. Milk, dairy fat, dietary calcium, and weight gain: A longitudinal study of adolescents. *Arch Pediatr Adolesc Med.* 159(6):543–50.

14. Adebamowo, CA, et al. 2005. High school dietary dairy intake and teenage acne. *J Am Acad Dermatol.* 52(2):207–14.

15. Feskanich, D, et al. 1997. Milk, dietary calcium, and bone fractures in women: A 12-year prospective study. *Am J Public Health.* 87(6):992–97.

16. Malosse, D, et al. 1992. Correlation between milk and dairy product consumption and multiple sclerosis prevalence: A worldwide study. *Neuroepidemiology.* 11(4-6):304–12.

17. Ceci, F, et al. 1989. The effects of oral 5-hydroxytryptophan administration on feeding behavior in obese adult female subjects. *J Neural Transm.* 76(2):109–17.

18. Cangiano, C, et al. 1998. Effects of oral 5-hydroxy-tryptophan on energy intake and macronutrient selection in non-insulin dependent diabetic patients. *Int J Obes Relat Metab Disord.* 22(7):648–54.

19. Bocarsly, ME, et al. 2010. High-fructose corn syrup causes characteristics of obesity in rats: Increased body weight, body fat and triglyceride levels. *Pharmacol Biochem Behav.* 97(1):101–6.

20. Tittelbach, TJ, et al. 2000. Post-exercise substrate utilization after a high glucose vs. high fructose meal during negative energy balance in the obese. *Obes Res.* 8(7):496–505.

21. Just, T, et al. 2008. Cephalic phase insulin release in healthy humans after taste stimulation? *Appetite.* 51(3):622–27. Epub 2008 May 10.

22. Liang, Y, et al. 1987. The effect of artificial sweetener on insulin secretion. 1. The effect of acesulfame K on insulin secretion in the rat (studies in vivo). *Horm Metab Res.* 19(6):233–38.

23. Davidson, TL, and SE Swithers. A Pavlovian approach to the problem of obesity. *Int J Obes Relat Metab Disord.* 28(7):933-35.

24. Sharma, RP, and RA Coulombe, Jr. 1987. Effects of repeated doses of aspartame on serotonin and its metabolite in various regions of the mouse brain. *Food Chem Toxicol.* 25(8)565–68.

25. Fowler, SP. 2005. *Diet soft drink consumption is associated with increased waist circumference in the San Antonio Longitudinal Study of Aging.* Webcast from the 65th annual scientific sessions of the American Diabetes Association, San Diego.

26. Blom, WA, et al. 2006. Effect of a high-protein breakfast on the postprandial ghrelin response. *Am J Clin Nutr.* 83(2):211–20.

27. Mierlo, CA, et al. 2003. Weight management using a meal replacement strategy: Meta and pooling analysis from six studies. *Int J Obes Relat Metab Disord.* 27(5):537–49.

28. University of Washington Study. 2002. Reported in *Integrated and Alternative Medicine Clinical Highlights.* Aug 4:1(16).

29. Rosenbaum, M, and RL Leibel. 2010. Adaptive thermogenesis in humans. *Int J Obes (Lond).* 34(Suppl 1):S47–S55.

30. Tsai, AG, and TA Wadden. 2005. Systematic review: An evaluation of major commercial weight loss programs in the United States. *Ann Intern Med.* 142(1):56–66.

31. University of Washington Study. 2002. Reported in *Integrated and Alternative Medicine Clinical Highlights.* Aug 4:1(16).

32. Donnelly, JE, et al. 2004. The role of exercise for weight loss and maintenance. *Best Pract Res Clin Gastroenterol.* 18(6):1009–29. (http://www.ncbi.nlm.nih.gov/pubmed/15561636)

33. Wing, RR, et al. 2005. Long-term weight loss maintenance. *Am J Clin Nutr.* 82(Suppl 1): 222S–225S. (http://www.ncbi.nlm.nih.gov/pubmed/16002825)

34. Pritzlaff, CJ, et al. 2000. Catecholamine release, growth hormone secretion, and energy expenditure during exercise vs. recovery in men. *J. Appl. Physiol.* 89(3):937–46.

35. Pacheco-Sánchez, M, and KK Grunwald. 1994. Body fat deposition: Effects of dietary fat and two exercise protocols. *J Am Coll Nutr.* 13(6):601–7.

 # MY FAVORITE BOOKS

*Adrenal Fatigue.* James L. Wilson, DC, ND, PhD

*Are You Tired and Wired?* Marcelle Pick, MSN, Ob/Gyn NP

*Breaking the Food Seduction.* Neal Barnard, MD

*Change Your Brain, Change Your Life.* Daniel G. Amen, MD

*Diet Wise.* Keith Scott-Mumby, MB, ChB, MD, PhD

*Digestive Wellness.* Elizabeth Lipski, PhD, CCN, CHN

*Eat, Drink and Be Gorgeous.* Esther Blum, MS, RD, CDN, CNS

*Healthier Without Wheat.* Stephen Wangen, ND

*Lights Out: Sleep, Sugar, and Survival.* T.S. Wiley

*Living Gluten-Free for Dummies.* Danna Korn

*Mindless Eating: Why We Eat More Than We Think.* Brian Wansink, PhD

*Naked Calories.* Mira Calton, CN and Jason Calton, PhD

*Nourishing Traditions: The Cookbook That Challenges Politically Correct Nutrition and the Diet Dictocrats.* Mary G Enig, PhD, Pat Connolly and Sally Fallon

*PACE: The 12-Minute Fitness Revolution.* Al Sears, MD

*Seeds of Deception: Exposing Industry and Government Lies About the Safety of the Genetically Engineered Foods You're Eating.* Jeffrey M. Smith

*Sexy Forever: How to Fight Fat after Forty.* Suzanne Somers

*The Blood Sugar Solution: The UltraHealthy Program for Losing Weight, Preventing Disease, and Feeling Great Now!* Mark Hyman, MD

*The Body Ecology Diet: Recovering Your Health and Rebuilding Your Immunity.* Donna Gates

*The Complete Idiot's Guide to Thyroid Disease.* Alan Christianson, NMD

*The Dietary Cure for Acne.* Loren Cordain, PhD

*The End of Overeating.* David Kessler, MD

*The 4-Hour Body.* Timothy Ferriss

*The Gut Flush Plan.* Ann Louise Gittleman, PhD, CNS

*The Metabolic Effect Diet.* Jade Teta, ND, CSCS and Keoni Teta, ND, Lac, CSCS

*The No Grain Diet.* Joseph Mercola, DO

*The 150 Healthiest Foods on Earth.* Jonny Bowden, PhD, CNS

*The Paleo Diet.* Loren Cordain, PhD

*The Paleo Solution: The Original Human Diet.* Robb Wolf

*The Primal Blueprint.* Mark Sisson

*The Protein Power Lifeplan.* Michael R. Eades, MD and Mary Dan Eades, MD (old but good information)

*The Real Food Diet Cookbook.* Dr. Josh Axe

*The Sleep Doctor's Diet Plan: Lose Weight Through Better Sleep.* Michael J. Breus, PhD

*The Smarter Science of Slim.* Jonathan Bailor

*The South Beach Wake-Up Call.* Arthur Agatston, MD

*The Whole Soy Story: The Dark Side of America's Favorite Food.* Kaayla T. Daniel, PhD, CCN

*Wheat Belly.* William Davis, MD

*Why You Can't Lose Weight.* Pamela Wartian Smith, MD, MPH

*Why We Get Fat.* Gary Taubes

 # VIDEOS

*Food Inc.* Robert Kenner, Director

*Got the Facts on Milk? The Milk Documentary.* T Colin Campbell, PhD and John A McDougall, MD

*King Corn.* Aaron Woolf, Director

# INDEX

weight loss, xx, 52, 225
  Cycle 2 and, 201
  Cycle 3 and, 225
  dropping the top 7 high-FI foods
    and, xix, xxi–xxii, 39
  exercise and, 225-35
  fast vs. slow, 41-42, 188
  five fundamentals for, 188-89
  maintenance tips, 220-22
  meal-replacement shakes and,
    215
  reducing stress and, 185
  7 pounds in 7 days, xxiv, xxvi,
    xxvii, 39, 44
  sleep and, 185
  10 pounds in 21 days, 186
  tracking guide and journal
    website, 188
  unsuccessful, xxi, 7, 225
  water and, 174
  weekly weigh-in, 220-21, 227, 235
whole grains, xix, xxi, xxiv, 6, 60-61,
    69, 163, 202. *See also* gluten
  gluten-free types, 69, 159
  Pasta Primavera, 284
  Roasted Vegetable Stuffed Pita,
    284
  sprouting, 164
  Turkey on Wheat, 285
  whole-wheat bread, 12
Willet, Walter, 95

## X

xylitol, 142, 183, 192, 253

## Y

yeast, 37, 126, 137, 205
yogurt, xvii, xxi, xxiv, 6, 12, 19,
    178
  coconut, 251
  eliminating, 37, 38, 39
  Greek-style, xix, 37, 99, 206
  Greek-Style (recipe), 290

## Z

zinc, 131, 158
zonulin, 24, 65
zucchini, 165
  Noodles, 300
  "the stoup," 248

# ABOUT THE AUTHOR

JJ VIRGIN, CNS, CHFS, is a highly regarded fitness and nutrition expert, public speaker, and media personality. *The Virgin Diet* has appeared on numerous bestseller lists, including the *New York Times, USA Today,* the *Chicago Tribune,* and the *Wall Street Journal.* JJ is also the bestselling author of *The Virgin Diet Cookbook, JJ Virgin's Sugar Impact Diet, JJ Virgin's Sugar Impact Diet Cookbook,* and *6 Weeks to Sleeveless and Sexy*, and the creator of the 4x4 Workout series.

Internationally recognized as an expert in helping people overcome weight-loss resistance—doing everything right according to current diet strategies but still not losing weight—JJ has helped hundreds of thousands of people finally lose weight by addressing food allergies, food sensitivities, and other food intolerances. Clients feel better in days and achieve fast, lasting fat loss when they drop the 7 highly reactive foods she has identified.

High-performance athletes, CEOs, and A-list celebrities seek out JJ to deliver the results they need and expect. She has provided nutrition and training programs for a wide variety of famous faces including Gene Simmons, Ben Stiller, Taj George, Jeanne Tripplehorn, Nicole Eggert, Tracie Thoms, Tamara Johnson-George, and "Superman" Brandon Routh.

JJ speaks at major integrative medical and consumer conferences, having shared the stage with Jack Canfield, Suzanne Somers, John Gray, Dr. Daniel Amen, and Brendon Burchard. A prominent media personality, she has appeared on PBS, *The Dr. Oz Show, The Rachael Ray Show, TODAY,* and *Access Hollywood.* She also cohosted two seasons of TLC's *Freaky Eaters,* and was the nutrition expert for two years on *Dr. Phil.*

JJ has been interviewed by numerous publications, including *Fox News Magazine, Woman's World, Health, LA Weekly, Cosmopolitan,* and the *Los Angeles Times,* and is also a frequent blogger for the Huffington Post, mindbodygreen, Prevention.com, Dr. Oz's Sharecare, and several other sites.

JJ is a lifelong learner and has completed forty graduate and doctoral courses in the areas of exercise science, nutrition, functional medicine, and psychology. She is a board-certified nutrition specialist through the American College of Nutrition, board-certified in holistic nutrition, and a certified health and fitness specialist through the American College of Sports Medicine.

Most important, JJ is the mother of two amazing teenage boys. One of them survived a near-fatal auto accident, and JJ used her knowledge, expertise, and peer network to take him from comatose to thriving. Every day JJ wakes up with gratitude to be able to spend another day with her children and to help more people live fuller lives by achieving better health. She lives with her family in Rancho Mirage, California.

For more information, please visit JJ at jjvirgin.com.